"Formulation and Optimization of Self Emulsifying Drug Delivery System for Effective Anthelmintic Therapy"

Acknowledgement

It is my privilege to utilize this golden moment and bow myself to acknowledge my mother Mrs. Sunita Mahajan, my father Mr. Chandrakant Mahajan and my wife Mrs. Rudrani for providing me an opportunity to pursue my higher education. It is indeed a privilege to express a deep sense of gratitude towards my sister Dr. Pooja and my brother Dr. Deepak; I thank them for their love, trust, patience unconditional support and encouragement to pursue my interests.

I take this opportunity to express my heart-felt & deep sense of gratitude with sincerity to my esteemed guide and mentor Dr. S. S. Pimple, Professor, Department of Pharmaceutics P.E. Society's Modern College of Pharmacy, Nigdi, Pune; I am in short of words to thank for her erudite guidance, faith and affection bestowed upon me throughout my research work. Words would fail to express the crucial nature of interactive help, I have received from for her cooperativeness, timely encouragement and invaluable suggestions, guidance in the assimilation of data of my dissertation work and her support in completing my assignment successfully.

I express my profound & deep sense of gratitude towards Dr. P. D. Chaudhari, Prof. & Principal, P.E. Society's Modern College of Pharmacy, Nigdi, Pune and Ex Dean, Faculty of Pharmaceutical Sciences, Savitribai Phule Pune University, Pune for his inspiring and instrumental role in providing me the research & infrastructure facilities at the college and encouragement for the successful completion of my project work.

I express my deep sense of gratitude towards Dr. V. V. Chopade, Professor, Department of Pharmaceutical Chemistry for solving my problems and providing timely help.

I express my immense sense of gratitude to all the other staff members, librarian Yadav madam and Rajendra Chaudhari, store *incharge Yogesh Patil, Vaishali Pansare Lab technicians Mahadev Kuchekar and Amol Sukal , C. K. Shinde, and all other lab attendees for helping me in finishing my project work successfully.*

I am grateful to Hemant, Nitin and Pavan including seniors whose creativities in the lab and their positive attitudes have directly or indirectly contributed in my work. I would always cherish the wonderful moments that we spend together.

I am grateful to thank to Micro Labs Pharmaceutical Ltd, Verna, Goa for providing gift samples.

Today, at the acme of my dissertation, I take this privilege and pleasure to acknowledge the contributions of many individuals who have been inspirational and supportive throughout my work and endowed me with the most precious knowledge to see success in my endeavour.

Above all, I thank God almighty for showering his infinite bounties, graces and mercies upon me. Once again I would like to thank all those mentioned & those that have unknowingly failed to mention in making this project a worthy endeavor.

Mr. Kiran Chandrakant Mahajan

CONTENTS

Sr. No.	Particulars	Page No.
i	List of Tables	i-iii
ii	List of Figures & Graphs	iv-v
iii	Abbreviations	vi-vii
iv	Abstract	-
1.	Introduction	1-26
2.	Literature Survey	27-34
3.	Need of Work	35-36
4.	Aim and Objectives	37
5.	Plan of work	38
6.	Drug and Excipients profile	39-51
7.	Materials and Methods	52-55
8.	Experimental work	56-73
9.	Results and Discussion	74-115
10.	Summary	116-117
11.	Conclusion	118
12.	Future Scope	119
13.	References	120-131
14.	Similarity Report	-
15.	Annexures	-

i. LIST OF TABLES

Table No.	Name of Table	Page No.
1.	Selection of drug according to BCS class	15
2.	Physicochemical properties of Praziquantel	39
3.	Physicochemical properties of Capmul MCM	40
4.	Physicochemical properties of Cremophor RH 40	41
5.	Physicochemical properties of Polyethylene Glycol 400	42
6.	Physicochemical properties of Aerosil 200	43
7.	Physicochemical properties of Neusilin US2	44
8.	Physicochemical properties of Doshion P-544 DS	45
9.	Physicochemical properties of Croscarmellose sodium	46
10.	Physicochemical properties of Sodium Starch Glycolate	46
11.	Physicochemical properties of Polyplasdone XL-10	47
12.	Physicochemical properties of Microcrystalline Cellulose	48
13.	Physicochemical properties of Povidone	49
14.	Physicochemical properties of Mannitol	50
15.	Physicochemical properties of Magnesium Stearate	51
16.	List of materials used in present work	52
17.	List of equipments/Instruments used in present work	54
18.	List of Software used	55
19.	Experimental range and level of independent variables	59
20.	The 2 factor CCD matrix experimental values	60
21.	Grades of emulsions	62
22.	Formulation of 3^2 factorial design for Praziquantel S-SEDDS	66
23.	Animals required for study	69
24.	List of Chemicals	70
25.	HPLC System Parameters	70
26.	Organoleptic properties of PZQ	74
27.	Absorbance data in Methanol	77
28.	Absorbance data in 6.8 pH phosphate buffer	78

29.	Absorbance data in 7.4 pH phosphate buffer	79
30.	Absorbance data in 0.1 N HCl	80
31.	Aqueous & pH dependent solubility data of PZQ	81
32.	Solubility of Praziquantel in various oils	82
33.	Solubility of Praziquantel in various surfactants and co-surfactants	83
34.	Emulsification ability of selected surfactants by using Capmul MCM as an oily phase	84
35.	Emulsification ability of selected Co-surfactants by using Capmul MCM as an oily phase and Cremophore RH40 as a Surfactant phase	84
36.	Evaluation of Thermodynamic stability and dispersion study of preliminary batches	85
37.	Characterization Parameters of P-L-SEDDS Formulations	87
38.	ANOVA for the Model	88
39.	Stability study data of F7 formulation of liquid SEDDS	94
40.	Adsorbent selection	95
41.	Powder characteristics of adsorbents after adsorption of liquid SEDDS	96
42.	Evaluation parameters for S-SEDDS tablets of Praziquantel	101
43.	Evaluation parameters of optimized formulation T3 during stability study	103
44.	Taste masking evaluation parameters	104
45.	% Recovery with Methanol at 100 ng/mL	105
46.	% Recovery with Methanol at 500 ng/mL	105
47.	% Recovery with Methanol at 1000 ng/mL	105
48.	% Recovery with Acetonitrile:Methanol at 100ng/mL	106
49.	% Recovery with Acetonitrile:Methanol at 500ng/mL	106
50.	% Recovery with Acetonitrile:Methanol at 1000 ng/mL	106
51.	% Recovery with Acetonitrile:Methanol:Water at 100ng/mL	106
52.	% Recovery with Acetonitrile:Methanol:Water at 500 ng/mL	107

53.	% Recovery with Acetonitrile:Methanol:Water at 1000 ng/mL	107
54.	Linearity concentration Vs Area Under Curve.	107
55.	Summary Table- Input Variable	108
56.	Summary Table- Output	109
57.	Pharmacokinetic calculation results	109
58.	The ratio of peak areas of Praziquantel to Praziquantel IS at various concentrations	110
59.	System suitability Parameters	111
60.	Intra-day precision (Day 1)	111
61.	Intra-day precision (Day 2)	111
62.	Intra-day precision (Day 3)	112
63.	Inter-day precision	112
64.	Intra-day Accuracy	112
65.	Intra-day Accuracy	112
66.	Method Precision	114
67.	Robustness parameter	114
68.	Robustness for Praziquantel	115

ii LIST OF FIGURES

Figure No.	Name of Figure	Page No.
1.	FTIR spectra of PZQ	75
2.	DSC thermogram of PZQ	75
3.	XRD spectra of PZQ	76
4.	Pseudo ternary phase diagram with Capmul MCM (oil) & Cremophore RH40/PEG400 (Smix) in different ratio A) 1:1 B) 2:1 C) 3:1	85
5.	3D response surface plots for the effect on variables on A) % Transmittance B) Globule size C) Self emulsification time D) % Drug release	88
6.	Counter plot for the effect of variables on A) % Transmittance B) globule size C) Self emulsification time D) % Drug release	89
7.	Photograph of optimized liquid SEDDS (F7)	90
8.	TEM image of optimized liquid SEDDS (F7)	91
9.	Globule size of optimized F7 formulation	92
10.	Zeta potential of optimized F7 formulation	92
11.	(a) *In-vitro* drug release profile of formulations F1 to F4 (b) *In-vitro* drug release profile of formulations F5 to F8	93, 94
12.	Earthworm in optimized liquid SEDDS (n=6)	95
13.	*In-vitro* dissolution study of drug from two different adsorbent	96
14.	SEM images of solid SEDDS	97
15.	DSC thermogram of (A) Praziquantel (B) Solid SEDDS Powder	98
16.	Infrared spectra of (A) Praziquantel (B) S-SEDDS mixture	99
17.	XRD spectra of (A) Praziquantel (B) Optimized S-SEDDS	100
18.	(a) : *In-vitro* drug release profile of formulations T1 to T5 (b) : *In-vitro* drug release profile of formulations T6 to T9	101, 102
19.	*In-vitro* drug release comparison of T3 & marketed sample (M)	102
20.	Chromatogram of STD Praziquantel and Diazepam IS solution	113
21.	Chromatogram of Praziquantel	113

ABSTRACT

The current study was aimed to develop and optimize a self emulsifying drug delivery system for pediatric patients to improve the oral bioavailability and solubility of the anthelmintic drug, Praziquantel (PZQ). The solubility of PZQ was estimated in various vehicles to select proper component combination. SEDDS was formulated from Capmul MCM (oil), Cremophore RH 40 (surfactant) and PEG 400 (co-surfactant). Central composite design was employed as statistical tool to optimize the formulation independent variables, X_1 (oil) and X_2 (surfactant: co-surfactant mixture ratio) of the SEDDS. Eight formulations composed of Capmul MCM, at Smix ratios (1:1, 2:1 & 3:1) were selected. The responses studied were % transmittance, globule size, self-emulsification time and % drug release. These variables had a significant effect on the responses studied. The % transmittance, globule size, self-emulsification time and % drug release of the optimized formulation were 99.62% ±0.18, 14.73±0.11 nm, 20.33±0.57 sec. and 98.65% ±0.06. Its zeta potential, polydispersity index, cloud point and % drug content were -44.43±0.23 mv, 0.117±0.0011, 87.7°C ± 0.60 and 99.64 % ±0.12. TEM study confirmed the uniform oil globules in the optimized liquid formulation. The optimized P-L-SEDDS (F7) has exhibit prominent anthelmintic activity on earthworms. The optimized liquid SEDDS formulation was formulated into free-flowing powder (S-SEDDS) by adsorption on the Neusilin US2 and compressed into tablets. S-SEDDS of Praziquantel with improved dissolution profile was successfully prepared by using Neusilin US2 as an adsorbent carrier. The solid state characterization of S-SEDDS powder was performed by using DSC, PXRD and SEM to investigate the physical nature of the drug. Doshion resin novel polymer is used for taste masking of drug.

The optimized S-SEDDS tablet T3 batch showed minimum disintegration time and maximum drug release. Further, the accelerated stability studies for 6 months revealed that optimized S-SEDDS tablets of Praziquantel (T3) were found to be stable without any significant change in physico-chemical properties.

In vivo pharmacokinetic activity in rats revealed that optimized S-SEDDS tablets (T3) had 2.14 folds higher bioavailability than marketed PZQ tablet and it produces rapid onset of action. The peak drug concentration (Cmax) of optimized S-SEDDS tablet T3 batch was approximately 1.76 fold higher than marketed tablet.

This novel dosage form might be a promising dosage form in the prevention of worm infections for pediatric patients. The developed S-SEDDS is a useful solid platform technology for improving solubility and oral bioavailability of PZQ.

1. INTRODUCTION

1.1. Oral Drug Delivery

Oral medicines are the usual method of treatment, because of their benefits, comfort in the administration of oral medicine, favored patients, economical efficacy and facility of large scale manufacture. Approximately 60% of currently available medicinal molecules are given via mouth. It is estimated nowadays that oral formulations account for about 90% of the worldwide market share of all human drug formulations. About 84% of best-selling medications, now worth 35 billion dollars, with an annual growth rate of 10%. Patients are often more likely than other parenteral methods to intravenous, subcutaneous, intramuscular and asthma injections. Oral wording is moreover; medicinal products given via oral procedure may cure pathological local illnesses such as colorectal abdomen, malignancies, infections, inflammation, bowel diseases, Gastroduodenum ulcers and reflux issues. [1-5]

However, it is difficult to create oral formulations primarily because to the physicochemical characteristics of medications, including low solubility and membrane permeability. The absorption of therapeutic drugs may also be reduced by the detection of a low degree of biological and chemical stability and physiological barriers such as pH, effect transportation and metabolism. In addition, certain medicines in the local region may lead to nausea and discomfort. Over the past four decades, numerous research were conducted to study medicine's absorption and transport, intestinal transportation, the GI tract microenvironment and GI fluid stability. Therefore, a comprehensive knowledge of physical chemistry, GI permentiality, biobarrers, pharmacokinetics and pharmacodynamics is a key aspect in the creation of oral drug delivery systems. The majority of oral medicines in the upper portions of the GI tract are absorbed through duodenum and jejunum. As the lower surface and stronger mucosal barrier of medicinal products in the stomach are smaller than the digestive tract than (thickness of 1.5 mm). [6-8] Epithelial cells are arranged in a single column. The lamella propria is projected to produce sandstones on the apical surface. A broad variety of pharmacological interactions and absorption occurs in about 5000–7000 microvilli per cell. Microvilli's qualities extend significantly to absorb the gut but also provide enzyme barrier because the border of the brush is rich in digesting enzymes.

GI-Lumen medicine is absorbed via a variety of layers of the epithelium, mucous membranes and blood or lymph capillary walls. A biologically adhesive system's long-term preservation allows for extended absorption both via local and systemic medication distributors. [9, 10]

Another aspect is the pharmaco-reduced pH of the GI fluid. The pH of the stomach fluctuates in fasting state with an average baseline pH of 2.18 ± 0.18. Consequently, stomach protection must be provided for medicines with poor stability under the acidic pH. Pepsine is pH-acidic active and quickly inactivated above 4. For digestion of most dietary proteins, this is essential. A adequate pH buffer may be disabled and the local pH can be increased by over 4. With enteric coatings such phthalates of acetate and methacrylate polymers, the protection against unstable medicinal products in acidic stomach pH conditions may be utilized. Duodenum is neutral as opposed to the stomach in a highly permeable portion of the intestine. [11-13]

For designing of the oral dosage form, the GI transit time is needed. The transit time of doses via the small intestine is consistent for people with a recognised 3 hour value and relies on the physical properties of dose forms such as density, size and food. However, the length of transit of the stomach varies and also bioavailables pharmaceutical compounds. In the end, this volatility may lead to unforeseen plasma levels and substantially decrease therapeutically. Two kinds of stomach motion are driven and mixed, which are mainly affected by feed or rapid circumstances and the sleeping cycle. Motility of peristalsis determines primarily the frequency and therefore the residence period following oral administration of a medication. In humans the bowel content has been determined to be 3 cm/min in the digestive system. In the higher parts of the digestive tract the transit rate is larger and decreases to the ileum. A 3-4 hour drug tablet is required for the whole gut. However, the transit time in the big bowel is much longer and relies on the fibre availability. It is believed that the trip through the big gut in healthy individuals takes 2-4 days. During the residence in the intestines, absorption of medicines not very solutions and which slowly diminish in digestive fluids is also replicable and medications which promote medicinal releases are employed. Transport carriers must also absorb transit or residence time of tiny medicine molecules since the maximal carrier density of these medicinal goods is favorably absorbed. Consequently, the quantity of absorption of medicines is directly influenced by the GI interval following oral administration. [14-19]

Food may affect the absorption, reduce, increase, delay or velocity of drugs. Food influences GI processes such as stomach emptying, bile acid production, pH changes and increased blood flow. In general, the co-administered meal uses pH dependent solutions for the treatment of hydrophobic medications or pharmaceuticals. [15, 20] Impressions of drug metabolism were linked to the inhibitory actions of Cytochrome P450 and to the suppression of these substances by metabolism.

The mouth, esophagus, stomach, duodenum, jejunum, ileum and colon may pass through the mucus membranes of the GI organs during medicinal use throughout the gastrointestinal system. The dissolution of a medication begins after a dose of oral fluids, after a dose-form aqueous medium penetration, which normally enables the solid dosage to breakdown into smaller particles. The next step is to mix into the drug molecule dissolving solution. The dissolving process has been examined. The mucosal membrane of the GI tract may be transported through a solution of medication molecules through a variety of methods, including passive diffusion and active transfer. The transcellular path includes the diffusion of the Liphospholipid across the intestinal enterocyte's cell membrane phospholipids. The path by which drugs pass via the tiny pores at the close intersection of the mucosal enterocytes is the transcellular route. Active drug transport is facilitated and split into an active drug and efflux pump inflow, by cell membrane transporters. The physico-chemical features of medicinal products and their attraction to various carriers determine the meaning of each mechanism. [21-26]

Transcellular pathways are the primary route of absorption for the smallest medication molecules. The transcellular trajectory in the paracellular pathway still absorbs the nonionised lipophilic drugs with a molecular weight more than 300 g/mol. Moreover, for the pharmaceutical products specified by the number of donors and recipients, hydrogen binding capacities should be less than 10, respectively. [27]

Flow across watery intercellular spaces by diffusion and convective volumes absorb medicinal chemicals during paracellular transfer. In general, this pathway mainly absorbs tiny hydrophilic molecules weighing less than 200 g/mol. In addition, the cationic molecules move free due to the total negative load on the intersectional complex of the intestinal epithelia. [28, 29]

The transport of carrier-mediated medicines through the apical membrane, typically in enterocyte cells, involves interactions with a protein carrier instead of passive medicinal dissemination. A number of transporters belonging to Adenosine Tryposphate (ATP) binding cassette (ABC) and solution conveyor (SLC) transporters are expressed in GI tube apical and basolateral membranes to supply or flow endogenous substances and xenobiotics. Absorption via this route is an energy expenditure and hydrolysis process involving ATP. A concentration gradient from a lower area of concentration to the higher concentration may be absorbed. Although many carriers are present in enterocytes, the absorption of drugs in the digestive system takes place mainly via just a restricted number of transporters. For instance, superfamily ABC operators use ATP to start transit and are known as main operating operators. Methotrexate, which is antagonist in follic acids, was absorbed through proximal intestine via the ABC-dépendant, proton-coupling folate transport/heme transporter protein. In contrast, mainly ion gradients (hydrogen, calcium and sodium ion gradients) are used by the SLC transporters (NA+/K+-ATPase and Na+/h+-ATPase). In contrast, enhanced medication absorption includes energy in a protein carrier but does not include energy. The drug concentration gradient as in passive diffusion is the primary driver of this absorption pathway. Classic examples of improved absorption include the intestinal absorption of glucose, folate and vitamin B12. [30-32]

1.2. Physicochemical Hurdles

GI medicinal products must be absorbed by releasing the dosage form. Dissolving medications must also be allowed to enter the intestinal wall. The main factors for the absorption of GI medicines are water solubility and epithelial membrane permeability, which provide the foundation for a BCS class-IV biopharmaceutical classification scheme for drug categorization. BCS is based on the dose strength solubility requirement, which can dissolve in a glass of water (capacity 250 ml) or in water with a pH of 2–7.5. Enterocytes are frequently referred as permeability through the apical membrane and rely on pharmaceutical items such as polarity, loading and lipophilicity. BCS Class-I drugs are highly soluble and permeable and provide excellent oral therapies. It is a difficulty for the oral administration of other BCS classes due to its poor solubility, low permeability and/or both (BCS Class-IV). By boosting their breakdown rate, BCS Class-II drugs may enhance their oral absorption capacity. [33-35]

In addition, drug metabolism may change its bioavailability, its solubility and its permeability. Wu and Benet thus developed the categorization scheme for biopharmaceutical products i.e. Biopharmaceutics Drug Disposition Classification System (BDDCS). The BDDCS offers information on dietary impact on the absorption, absorption, removal and transport of medicinal products. The drug permeability is according to the BDDCS according to the main elimination pathway. BDDC Class-1 there are no anticipated to be significant metabolism in major interactions with high solubility. The amount of bioavailability of such products should therefore not be altered by high fat meals. High-fat meals nevertheless delay aspiration and reduce absorption, increasing Tmax. The non-highly soluble and metabolized BDDCS Class-2 medicines may be susceptible to the substantial transport effects and in particular, their insolubility, impacts of effluent carrier systems. Since efflux pumps such as PGP carriers are stopped in the intestines, their biomass availability may increase with high fat meals. Dosage forms that substantially enhance BDDCS class-2 solubility may minimise or eliminate fatty meals effects and mainly limit further interactions between medication carriers. Due to their poor permeability, the impact of absorbed transport is especially sensitive for BDDCS class-3 drugs. Fatty meals may decrease many pharmaceutical products bioavailability by reducing bowel absorption carriers. The major implications of this mechanism nevertheless rely on the level and relative affinity of the substratum to carrier blocks in medicine carriers (influx and efflux). This may increase the bioavailability of drugs unexpectedly or have no effect. The impact of fatty foods on medicines absorbed in Class-4 of BDDCS is hard to anticipate since interaction combinations between Class-2 and Class-3 is conceivable. The combination of increased solubility of a GI medicine and efflux transport inhibition is the main source of such effects nevertheless in fatty meal effects, thereby enhancing the bioavailability. [36-40]

1.3. Biochemical Barriers

Digestive enzymes of the pancreas, along with those produced from the colon intestinal flora, are located mostly in the lower portion of the gastrointestinal system (lipsasis, amylase, peptidases and chymotrypsin). Intra-cyte and intra-brush metabolism on the enterocyte surface are also enzymes inside the membrane of the border of the brush and the first-pass metabolism. The brush border is mostly metabolized in the small intestine. Isomaltases, alkaline phosphatase, sucrose and other peptidases are used to support the metabolism of the brush borders. The metabolism of the first pass may reduce oral absorption. [36]

Mainly phase-I enzymes, including cytochrome P450 (CYP3A4), comprise enterocytes. Metabolism intracellular to enterocytes occurs. Phase-II Multiple conjugates enzymes linked to sulphate and glucuronidation. Although the gut epithelium is a location for pre-absorption of metabolism, average drugs like aspirin may be given. In addition, besides the intestine, the main metabolic barrier is the liver metabolism of the first pass. [37]

Transporters of the mucous membrane may be divided into two types: absorbent and efflux carriers, transporters of endogenous substances, and transporters of medicines. In membrane transporters the absorption, disposal and biodisposal of oral drugs are major factors. The primary transport vehicles that allow the transportation of medicinal product into the cell are held by the SLC superfamily and by efflux carriers, by the ABC superfamily. Efflux transporters have been extensively expressed in liver and intestines such as the bile-salt exportation pump (BSEP), p-gp, MRP1-6 and BCRP. Most of these membrane carriers use ATP for concentration gradient pump substrates. In addition, CYP3A4 co-locates P-gp in the mature enterocytes and overlaps the specification of the substratum. Consequently, most substratum medicines may be metabolized before re-absorption to the cells by pumping P-gp from their enterocyte into the lumen, increasing their CYP3A4 exposure. The bioavailability of many drugs is restricted by this method. It may also lead to interactions with medicines, particularly when pharmaceuticals are used to inhibit P-gp or CYP3A4. [41-44]

1.4. Strategies for Improving Oral Drug Delivery

The development of oral medicines with low solubility is difficult to comprehend. Drug solubility is a major role in hydrophobic medications poor oral bioavailability. Dietary consequences, stomach discomfort, delayed effects, lack of sufficient and significant variation between and between individuals, are additional reasons for the poor bioavailability of hydrophobic medicines. For the development of poorly soluble medicinal formulations the formulation issues involving tensile selection, particle size reduction and salt selection must be properly addressed. A mixture of surfactants has traditionally been used to improve oral absorption. Tensile substances are hydrophilic, with a hydrophilic tail with drug molecules, which reduce the contact stress, both hydrophilic and lipophilic surfaces. Surfactants improve pharmaceutical bioavailability by opening close intracellular joints over a period of time via several means, including increased solubility and permeability. Tensile substances may continue to be a security issue at greater levels and must be properly handled. Additional methods such as micro-nanonization may also increase the bioavailability of medicines significantly. These methods significantly decrease the particle size of medicinal products and enhance their dissolving rate. [43-46]

Because of its simple management, simplicity and economical, straight forward design, oral route is the most commonly used method to medication. Some 40% of new drugs have poor solubility in water, leading to restricted bioavailability, substantial heterogeneity in subject and topic matter and inadequate dose proportionality. Many medicines also impede oral administration due to their high hydrophobicity. Consequently, adequate formulations should enhance the solubility and bioavailability of such therapeutic compounds. Self-emulsifying medical goods were recently shown to be a major interest in enhancing the availability of poor medicines in oral biology.

SEDDS is an isotropic drug combination, which, when diluted with physiological fluid, produces excellent quality emulsion and liquid droplets. During the whole process, the medication is dissolved and the absorption of the crystalline hydrophobia is often delayed. The distribution strategy depends on stability, production techniques, content interaction and the storage temperature of the capsule. In the SEDDS self-emulsification process is controlled by a mixture of the oil surfactants. All variables include oil structure, surfactant level, oil/surfactant ratio and temperature autoemulsification. SEDDS is easy to manufacture. The number of SEDDS researchers has steadily increased. Solid SEDDS produced in powder by solidification of liquid self-emulsifiers are the most common SEDDS. These S-SEDDS were generated by means of extrusion, wet granulation or sorption in a high shear mixer for solid carriers, integrating the liquid mixture into a liquidator, respectively. Their capacity to improve the oral bioavailability of medications with poor absorption increases their rate of dissolution or delivers the drug in solution form throughout the gastrointestinal tract, since dissolution is usually the limiting rate. [47-52]

- Protection against enzymatic hydrolysis.
- Improvement in oral bioavailability.
- High thermodynamic stability.
- High drug solubilization capability.

The poor conformity of their lipid content was the most troublesome microemulsion. Because of its high water content, neither hard gelatin nor soft gelatin can encapsulate a micro-emulsion. An alternate form has to be converted to anhydrous autoemulsifying systems for drug administration due to the low-dose SEDDS (SEDDS).

The lipid-based formulations include a natural or synertic composition, solid or fluid and co-surfactants of isotropic composition. The formula of SEDDS is the same. When they are introduced with aqueous medium they undergo self-emulsification for O-W nanoemulsion or microemulsions. (e.g. gastrointestinal fluids). Therefore, SEDDS are generally termed auto-nano-emulsifying drug delivery systems based on the kind of dispersion produced after dilution (SNEDDS).

The SEDDS showed that, via various underlying processes, in particular the class-II mechanisms of classification systems, the oral bio-availability of poor-soluble medicines may be enhanced. The most often studied causes were increased solubility of medicines.

Components of lipidic SEDDS promote Lipoprotein/Chylomicron synthesis, increasing medicinal absorption. The ultra-fine droplets in the emulsion resulting from a wide region of contact with the gastrointestinal (GI) membranes. The biometric effects of the several components used in the SEDDS formulation contributed substantially to the greatly increased bioactivity of pharmaceutical goods. Strict opening of the junction and increased membrane fluidity through the high concentration of SEDDS comprise these bioactive effects. It has also been seen as effective techniques for stimulating the intestinal lymph route and inhibiting pumps for the use of intestinal medications (P-gp and CYP3A4) to enhance oral delivery of P-gp substrates, and bypass the metabolism of the intestinal and liver primary hand. P-gp is the most extensively distributed ATP transmembrane transporter throughout the body and is an energy-dependent membrane-like protein. P-gp reduces the accumulation of endogenous chemicals and xenobiotics by bringing them back to the extracellular region. Thus, intestinal p-gp carriers, by decreasing their bowel absorption from substrate treatment, decrease their oral bioavailability. In addition, P-gp transport over-expression is indicated by the development of multi-drug resistance (MDR) in many distinct human cancer types. Several methods to decrease P-gp activity have thus been developed to enhance oral bioavailability in P-gp substrates and to reverse MDR in tumor cells. Among these methods nanocarriers have been extensively studied. P-gp substrates in nanocarriers are shielded against pre-termed releases and biological interactions. They regulate medicinal tissue dispersion and favorably accumulate in the tumor tissue. The oral bioavailability of p-gp medicinal products and reverse MDR in tumor cells across different nanocarreries has been extensively investigated by SEDDS.

It is noteworthy that both hydrophobic and hydrophilic medicines are more orally accessible due to the unique mix of SEDDS functions. The oral provision of protein and genetic materials is essential because of its hydrophilic nature and high molecular weight. We address the latest advances with regard by using SEDDS to enhance oral bioavailability of P-gp substrates, reverse MDR in tumor cells and therapy of oral protein and genetics. The aim of this project is to highlight a unique combination of SEDDS characteristics which improve the oral usage of target medicines via multifunctional delivery systems. [51-59]

In the last 20 years, SEDDS has carefully examined the entire control of P-gp mediated substratum efflux. The ability of SEDDS to suppress P-gp activities depends mostly on excipients included in the formulation of a known P-gp inhibitor. The most frequent excipients used for P-gp inhibition in SEDDS are nonionic surfactants. SEDDS is taken into account. Cremophor EL, Cremophor RH40, Labrasol, Transcutol P, Tween 80 are among the most common uses. The HLB value and hydrophobic domain structure for a particular surfactant are the foundation for inhibitory p-gp activity. The HLB levels of surfactants are not obviously related to P-gp-inhibition action. Structural links should be made to hydrophobic surfactant molecules to decrease P-gp activity by the hydrophobic hydrophilic side chains. [60]

In contrast to its separate components, SEDDS is more effective and efficient *in vivo*. A number of SEDDS formulations may enhance its inhibitory p-gp action. In ultra-fine emulsion droplets, P-gp picking protects against the identification of GI pathological P-gp efflux pumps. SEDDS also allows co-management of several excipients close to the GI epithelium. SEDDS formulations may also contain pharmaceutical excipients that have shown inhibition of P-gp (eg. Curcumin). [61,62]

On the other hand, the consequences of over-expressed P-gp transport in tumor cells provide a considerable barrier to cancer treatment. The over-expression of SEDDS by P-gp transporter in tumor cells for the elimination of MDRs is thoroughly investigated. The SEDDS allows several chemical therapies to be combined via different routes in the same vector in order to provide synergistic effects against cancer. SEDDS may be used by different antioxidants to reduce oxidative stress in cancer cells. It's awesome & it is very interesting. [63-65]

In almost every area of medicine, protein therapy plays an important role. These methods of delivery, however, contradict the widespread use of protein treatment through a parenteral route linked to poor patient compliance. The development of non-invasive protein treatment methods gives rise to major concerns. For the administration of protein treatment, oral methods were widely investigated. Unfortunately, a range of obstacles, such as acidic environments in your stomach, degraded GI enzymes, mucus barrier and cellular inappropriate penetration; jeopardize an oral provision of protein or peptide therapies. Various methods of overcoming these limitations were proposed. As potential suppliers of protein and peptide therapy orally SEDDS have been widely studied. During hydrophilic macromolelecular therapy for example, a number of surfactants and oils are beneficial to enhance penetration of the formulation of SEDDS. The extremely fine gout offers a wide area for quick entry of digestion. Protein against water breakdown is protected by the anhydrous SEDDS structure. SEDDS assist to improve the oral bioavailability of the loaded protein. Therapeutic products with additional bioactive effects, including tight junction openings and increased absorption from lymph. The hydrophilic nature of protein therapy is questioned by SEDDS. Consequently, before integrated in the SEDDS preconcentration, the lipid solubility's of protein treatment should be enhanced. This may be done in many methods, such as the double-emulsion and hydrophilic or co-solvent solvents hydrophobic ion-packaging and chemical modifications to the molecule of peptides. [65-67]

1.5. Definition of SEDDS

SEDDS are ideally isotropic oils and surfactants which include cosurfactants/co-solvents, which spontaneously emulsify in order to create fine oil as water emulsion when they are applied under mild restlessness during the water phase. The use of triglyceride oils with a medium chain and lower hazardous nonionic surfactants has recently been developed for SEDDS. These methods produce fine emulsions or microemulsions, due to stomach movement, during gastrointestinal tract (GIT) peroral delivery. Fine oil droplets would quickly travel into the stomach and distribute the medication throughout the gastrointestinal system and minimise the inconveniences that occur in interaction between bulk pharmaceutical components and the intestinal wall. The basic characteristics are that, compared with the transparent microemulsion SEDDS produces opaque emulsions between 100 nm and 300 nm droplets size. The oil level in SMEDDS in comparison with 40-80% in SEDDS is likewise under 20%. Possible benefits include improved oral dose-cutting bioavailability, increased consistency of time patterns for medication absorption, a selective GIT-specific drug screen and drug safety. SEDDS are isotropic mixes containing one or more hydrophilic surfactants and natural or produced oil. These produces oil after proper turbulence and dilution from binary compound media like GI in the emulsion of water. The device produces oil in the water emulsion. The motility of the intestine makes in situ emulsification and restlessness possible. These formulations are available for simple administration and accurate doses in soft and hard gelatin capsules. If an oral solution is possible, it should first be emulsified into a glass of water before administration of SEDDS. [68-73]

1.6. Enhancement of Oral Bioavailability [74-78]

The bioavailability of low-solution medicines is a major issue with absorption that influences the rate of dissolution. In order to convey the physical phenomena of the binary intestinal compound and of the membrane bordering an absorbing brush, SEDDS capability to transport drugs to GIS with a higher surface is soluble and low-emulsified to carry highly effective drugs that lead to enhanced bioavailability.

1.6.1. Scale-up

The bioavailability of poorly soluble medicines may be a significant problem because of the absorption that influences the dissolving rate. With a solution-limited and low-emulsified surface area in a more specific condition and enable increased biological availability, SEDDS may transport the physical phenomenon of the binary gut chemistry and brush-absorbent membrane.

1.6.2. Effects of food

There are significant inter and intra-subject absorption differences in many medications, which contribute to poorer drug performance and non-compliance for patients. Diet affects the therapeutic effectiveness of a medicine in the body. For such drugs, SEDDS may be helpful. Meals do not affect SEDDS functionality and SEDDS offers the replicability of plasma profiles in numerous investigations.

1.6.3. GIT enzyme hydrolysis

The ability of SEDDS to transport and maintain macromolecules including peptides, hormone substrates and inhibitors is a distinct feature of conventional drug delivery systems. Cholinesterase bowel hydrolysis may be inhibited using polysorbate 20 in the case of the microemulsion formulations. These are energy-free or hot-free systems that may be utilized in thermolabile drugs such as peptides.

1.6.4. The impact of lipoid digestion

SEDDS does not affect lipolysis, emulsifying with the aid of digestive fluids, the action of the gland lipase duct, or mixed particle formations, as in other lipid-base techniques for medicinal administration. The SEDDS seems not to have been digested completely before absorption since the drug's microemulsion can permeate only unaggregated glycoprotein.

1.6.5. Improved capacity for medication loading

Because of its usually limited solubility in natural lipids, but considerably greater in amphiphillic surfactants, co-surfactants and co-solvents for water-soluble drug products with intermediate partition coefficients (2 logP > 4) SEDDS has a larger capacity than conventional lipid solutions.

1.6.6. Advantages of SEDDS [79-82]

1. SEDDS offer, in addition to providing hydrophobic solubility benefits as emulsions, solves the emulsion stacking issue after a lengthy sitting. SEDDS are often kept only because they form part of a stable thermodynamic system.
2. SEDDS microemulsions thermodynamically stable and transparent. The main

difference between tiny emulsions and regular emulsions is the particle size of the droplets. Micro-emulsive droplets measure between 0.2 and 10 nm, whereas SEDDS-generated micro-emulsion droplets measure 2 and 100 nm. Since the particle size is small, the whole area available for absorption and dispersion is much greater than in a solid formulation and may be absorbed and absorbed more quickly. This will lead to an increase in the bioavailability of the medication.

3. SEDDS offers hard gelatin capsules, soft gelatin capsules and tablets. Emulsions are employed exclusively as oral solutions, on the other hand.
4. Emulsions cannot be autoclaved because the reverse section temperature is needed whereas SEDDS are often autoclaved.

1.7. Approaches of self-emulsifying drug delivery systems [83-85]

The self-emulsifying drug delivery systems (SEEDS) are oil and tensile emulsifying mixtures that mimic moderate turbulence in the emulsion of the gastrointestinal tract. Ideally, with co-solvents they are isotropic. Before embedding in dosage forms for the oral unit, hydrophobic medicine is usually dissolved. A fine emulsion is produced when self-emulsifier formulations are mixed carefully and exposed to the binary compound media. Due to restricted space inside the oil stretching region, the emulsions are stable, the droplet dispersion is decreased and oil droplet polarity is low. After oral administration of SEDDS, the biological movement of the body and consequently of the gut allows for the necessary restructuring to self-emulsify, which can be easily seen with soft-gelatin capsules. Compared to previous oral preparations, the amount and rate of oleophilic chemicals taken in by autoemulsified products have substantially risen. The absorption of medicinal drugs in the mouth may be improved by SEDDS and SMEDDS.

1.8. Biopharmaceutical Point of view [86-88]

More information has been obtained on the potential to improve biological availability of water-soluble fluids and/or food medicinal products and may be recommended by interested readers. While the exact processes do not appear, lipids should improve bioavailability via a variety of methods, including:

1. Gastrointestinal transit time changes which will lead to a delayed delivery and extended shutdown.
2. Effective luminary drug solubility is growing. Favor bile salt (BS) and endogenous bile

lipids such as phospholipids (PL) and cholesterol (CH) in the GI tract are present, resulting to the production of bile micelles and the increase of solubility of the GI tract. Interconnected lipides in these BS structures lead either directly (if polar) or via digestion to the enlargement of the micellular structures and to the increase of solubilization ability.

3. Transportation stimulation of the intestinal lymph. Lipids may enhance lymphatic transport and enhance bioavailability for very lipophilic therapeutic compounds via direct or indirect reduction of first pass metabolism.
4. The biochemical barriers function of the GI tract changes. The P-glycoprotein efflux pump shows that certain lipids and surfactants adversely affect enterocyte metabolism and reduce the function of the bowel efflux conveyor.
5. The physical barriers function of the GI tract changes. Several combinations have shown enhanced permeability of fluids, lipids and surfactants. On the other hand, the bioavailability of most water-soluble and lipophilic medications is regarded to represent a major barrier to passive intestinal permeability.

1.9. Drug absorption by fluid delivery [89, 90]

A log of P more than 5 and triglyceride solubility over 50 mg/ml should be used for lymphatic transfer. In order to perform clinical and pharmacokinetic research on pediatric patients, appropriate age formulations must be developed. According to the PDREA and the Pediatric Research Equity Act, the FDA requires pediatric clinical studies. A Pediatric Survey Plan (PIP) is needed for the European Medicine Evaluation Agency (EMEA) before new marketing licensing medicines are submitted (EMEA 2011). The World Health Organization has started an effort to support the development, under the name "Make Child Size Medicines," of appropriate pediatric formulations. The reflecting document on pediatric medicine offers information on optimum formulations of patient ages (EMEA 2005). Pediatric and the elderly find it difficult to sweep big pills and capsules. Multidrug usage by older individuals is used in many treatments, including diabetes, hepatitis and renal failures, diseases in coronary heart, arthritis, impairments of the vision and neurologic issues. Older individuals are hard to swallow big tablets and to grab small medicines and to misbehave the old ones, memory loss and co-measurement. For older individuals, adjustments in dosage may be required depending on their physiological condition and condition. Flexible formulations may be chosen for pediatric or geriatric patients, in accordance with the WHO recommendations FDA and EMEA. Suitable medication delivery methods are required to provide effective therapy for pediatric and geriatric patients. Age groupings and proposed types of dose for children, adults and seniors. The fluids and syrups, suspensions, drops, granules, multiparticle powders, chewables, oral dissolving tablets (ODT) and the capsules of traditional and oral dissolving tablets (ODT) are now available in scatterable tablets and capsules. Currently available are oral disintegrating tablets and capsules. Due to the market size of the majority of individuals, the majority of dosage forms have been developed and produced worldwide in adult patients. Since young individuals are not properly formed, adult medicines are required.

In order to improve its solubility and oral bioprocessing, the objective of this research was to develop stable self-emulsifying medicines for low water soluble drug Praziquantel. This leads to improved compliance with pediatrics patients with reduced dosage frequency. Efficiency and acceptance also depends on the safe masking of formulations for pediatric usage. In juvenile and geriatrically adjusted compliance, the disagreeable, bitter, or astringent taste of pharmaceutical components is important. For efficient taste masks only dry powders, solids, granules and multi-particulate formulations may be employed since the substance is a fluid-formulated solvent.

Many techniques of flavor masking are used in oral formulations. The flavor masking method used has an impact on the pharmacological variables pKa, solubility, size and taste of particles. Depending on the taste and dose of medicine, masking procedures such as altering the pH, various salts or forms of drugs, complexing of ion exchange resin (IER) and cyclodextrins (CD) as well as a coating matrix or barrier may be utilized for the usage of polymers and lipid materials. Using a combination of flavor masking/sweetener, the whole taste masking may be done and the formulas in pediatric patients are made more tastefully. Doshion polymers are also employed to disguise the flavor of pediatric medications, which is of great benefit to the acceptance of them. [91-93]

1.10. Selection of SEDDS Medication Candidate

Bioavailability is described as linked functions of permeability and solubility of the medicinal component in biopharmaceutical categorization scheme (BCS). When packed into lipid solubilization excipients, BCS compounds of category 'II' or low water solutions and strong membrane permit likely to exhibit a substantial improvement in biodiversity. BCS helps identify therapeutic substances which are bioavailable and which may be improved using oral lipid formulations. When utilized correctly, lipid formulations may enhance the bioavailability of medical medicinal products in all BCS categories.

Table 1. Selection of drug according to BCS class

BCS Class	Aqueous Solubility	Membrane Permeability
I	High	High
II	Low	High
III	High	Low
IV	Low	Low

By using the lipid solution in BCS class-II increases the bioavailability of the gastrointestinal system by removing barriers and dissolving low water solubility's. The exact procedures may be transported via the mixed micellar phase of bile salt to absorb the gut epithelium.

Lipids is able to improve bioavailability by decreasing the bowel effluence of p-glycoprotein transporters, reducing the metabolism of the bowel associated with the cytochrome enzyme and altering bowel fluid to increase permeability. Lipids may carry lipid-soluble medications to the lymph in the bowel and therefore hinder the first-pass hepatic therapy quickly reaching a systemic circulation. [94, 95]

1.11. Excipients employed in SEDDS [96, 97]

For the expanded release of oil, surfactants, co-surfactants, co-solvent and sometimes polymers, SEDDS formulations are employed. SEDDS is based on the surfactant by using type of the automated emulsification technique. All of them contribute to the process and effectively emulsify specific combinations of medicinal excipients, by oil and surfactant concentrations, oil/surfactant and self-emulsion temperature.

1. Oils

Oil has the potential to solve the right levels of poorly water-soluble medications, improve digestive absorption, and enhance lipophilic transportation through the lymph system. This depends on the molecular structure of a triglyceride. The long and medium chain triglyceride oils used to produce self-emulsifying compositions with different degrees of saturation. Food oils which signal the development of SEDDS are also available. SEDDS are seldom used or selected due to lipophilic dissolving problems. Plant oils have frequently been used, changed or hydrolyzed as emulsification is appropriate, oral administration is permitted and pharmaceutical solubility is enhanced. Their formulation is comparable to those of natural intestine digestion products and their physiological advantages. The standard medium-chain triglyceride oil effectively substitutes new semisynthetic, amphiphilic and surfactant by self emulsifying compounds.

2. Surfactants

The hydrophilic group may classify the surfactant molecules in the molecules. The four main surfactants are;

- **a)** Anionic
- **b)** Cationic
- **c)** Ampholytic (also called Zwitter ionic surfactants)
- **d)** Non-ionic

Non-ionic surfactants are the surfactants with strong hydrophilic-lipophilic balance for self-emulsifying systems (HLB). Emulgators include various polyglycolyzed and monoolylated polyoxyethylene glycerides, both solid and liquid (Tween 80). Natural surfactants are less dangerous than synthetic surfactants, but their low auto-emulsification capacity does not recommend them. Typically, the surfactant concentration for stable SEDDS is ranging from 30 to 60% w/w. The surfactant content should be adjusted since excessive quantities of surfactants may induce GI discomfort.

The surfactant used in SEDDS should have high HLB and hydrophilicity in the aquatic environment, such that o/w droplets are quickly generated and dispersed immediately (good self-emulsifying capabilities). In order to efficient absorption the precipitation in the GI lumen of drug molecules must be avoided and the drugs must continue to be solubilized as long as feasible at the absorption site. Surfactants are an amphiphilic agent that may be resolved by a broad range of hydrophobic substances or solutions. SEDDS are produced utilizing oil and lipid mixes.

The size of the droplet and the amount of surfactant used are linked. In some cases, an increase in the surfactant concentration may lead to smaller medium-sized droplets. A mixture of saturated polyglycolyzed C8-C10 glycerides may be used. In certain cases though, the medium size may contribute to greater amounts of surfactants. More water in the oil droplet may explain this conduct by an increase in the tensile content, causing the oil droplet to expel in the aqueous phase.

Historically, to increase permeability, tensile and surfactant compounds are employed. Some of the following excipients may be used to create oral SEDDS. The main advantage of these excipients is that they are generally allowed to be used on oral medicines.

3. Co-Surfactants

Given that a high concentration of tensile surfactant is required in order to properly reduce the interface tension, the co-surfactant is used to minimise the concentration of tensile surfactant. Co-Surfactants enable the interface layer to adapt in a variety of compositions along with surfactants to the different curvatures necessary for micro-emulsion. The effective production of SEDDS and the solubilization into SEDDS requires an adequate selection of the surfactant and surfactant products.

A co-surfactant is usually used with an HLB of 10-14. Significant quantities of lipid pharmaceutical or hydrophilic surfactants, such as ethanol and polyethylene glycol, may be dissolved and orally safe and thus can be used with SEDDS as a co-surfactant. In contrast, alcohols and other volatile co-solvents are not suitable for soft/hard gelatin capsules to evaporate, resulting in precipitation. On the other hand, lipophilic dissolving potential has been decreased by formulations without alcohol. As a consequence, a careful choice of components is required to synthesize effective SEDDS.

4. Co- Solvents

Co-solvents are water miscible organic soluble agents that are used to increase water solubility or the chemical stability of a medicinal substance in liquid medical formulations. Many orders in addition to their water solubility may enhance the solution ability of a non-polar medication by increasing co-solvents. Core solvents are a simple and potentially efficient technique for the production of high medication concentrations in non-polar formulations. The co-solvency approach may improve solubility and chemical stability via a number of methods. When the medication is susceptible to hydrolysis degradation, co-solvents may help to replace all or some water. On the other hand, the co-solvent may enhance the solubility of a drug by reducing the transitional status of the reactants. The transition state is more polar than the reaction, yet it works.

Organic solvents such as ethanol, propylene glycol (PG) and polyethylene glycol (PEG) are ideal for oral administration and can dissolve large numbers in the production of SEDDS in optimum condition. These solvents may also work in the microemulsion system as co-surfactants. In conventional shells of soft gelatin, alcohols and other volatile co-solvents are inconvenienced to evaporate into precipitation of medications. This leads to developing formulations without alcohol, but these may have limited their capacity to dissolve lipophilic medicines.

1.12. SEDDS Formulation

SEDDS is simple to manufacture because just the appropriate combination of oil and surfactant needs to be combined. Dosage sizes such as soft gelatin capsules filled with liquid or hard gelatin capsules with a gelatin ring that prevent leakages may be administered to pre-concentrate.

1.12.1. Factors Affecting Formulation of SEDDS [61]

1. Nature of the oil/surfactant pair and surfactant concentration.
2. Surfactant concentration and oil/surfactant ratio;
3. Surfactant to co-surfactant ratio.
4. Temperature at which self-emulsification occur.

1.12.2. Mechanism of Self-Emulsification process [56]

Reiss says that self-emulsification occurs when the entropy is higher than the energy needed for the dispersion surface to be increased. The necessary energy to develop a new interface between the water and the oil phases determines the energy for a typical emulsion. The two emulsion phases split the interface and therefore the free energy of the system over time. The following may be represented as equation 1:

$$\Delta G = \sum N \pi r^2 \sigma \qquad \text{----------------------} \ (1)$$

Where,

ΔG is the process-related free energy (ignorance of the mixing free energy),

N is the number of droplets of radius r,

σ denotes the interfacial energy.

1.12.3. Applications of SEDDS System [41, 91]

1. Improvement in drug solubility & drug bioavailability
2. Super saturable SEDDS
3. Protection against biodegradation

4. Herbal drugs and traditional medicine SEDDS

5. Solid SEDDS

1. Drug solubility and bioavailability enhancement

The lipid phase interacts readily and forms a micro-o/w emulsion with water on SEDDS devices. In dissolved condition, this o/w emulsion gout delivers the medication molecule to GIT and is easily absorbed.

2. Super saturable SE system

The surfactant and the addition of HPMC and other inhibitors of cellulose polymer precipitation may be maintained in a super-saturated condition for many years. These polymers prevent the medicine from crystallizing and allow it to remain in a super-saturated state. There are no surfactant side effects with these formulations and they provide fast absorption of the medicine. Excess surfactants irritate the gastrointestinal system. The low-surfactant SEDDS formulation has an improved toxicity and safety profile compared to the conventional SEDDS.

3. Defence from Biodegradation

Due to the pH or enzyme failure of the stomach, some medications in the biological system may be destroyed. Acetic salicylic acid is produced by gastrointestinal hydrolysis at pH acid; nevertheless, the deterioration is avoided by the SE system and its plasma concentration profile exceeds commercial formulation.

4. SEDDS of Herbal Medicine

The SEDDS technique used a number of natural medications. Silybin has been shown to protect liver cells against adverse effects such as stress, smoking, drinking habits, contaminants and products harming their liver, but its water solubility is poorly bioavailable by oral means. Its bioavailability has increased four times in the SE dose form. The Alzheimer's effects are all seen in cerebrovascular, antiischaemic, neuroprotective, antioxidant, cardiovascular and anti-disease extracts of Ginkgo Biloba. Dissolution, oral absorption and developing concentration period profiles for the less soluble active ingredients of Ginkgo biloba were improved by using the SEDDS formulation.

5. Solid SEDDS

SEDDS are fluid formulations that should be poured into SGCs, however certain manufacturing problems occur. Solidity of liquid formulas may thus be a feasible alternative. Solid formulations consist of powder, pellets and granules, such as tablets and capsules.

1.12.4. Drawbacks of SEDDS

SEDDS is characterized by two disadvantages: chemical and surfactants instability. GIT is irritated by the high tensile content of self-emulsifying goods (30-60%). Excipients of soluble, insoluble and tensile waters may all be employed as excipients solubilizers. Grinding is a common way of reducing the part of pharmaceutical business, but produces heat, sound and vibration power. It's a cooled, low-heat sample technique that may be utilized in a variety of biological and unstable chemicals (plants, animals). Melting leads, however, to mechanical activation of the crystalline solid and the production of energy, which may cause physical and chemical changes and reduce its efficiency.

1.12.5. Approaches to Self Emulsifying Drug Delivery Systems [98, 99]

The method of self-emulsifier drug delivery provides advantages in overcoming drug solubility and absorption difficulties, but it remains a challenge to obtain the drug as it stands. The most frequent type of medicine is the oral dosage, and lipid formulation provides much flexibility because liquids, semisolids or solids may be the form of oral administration. On the contrary, traditional systems with self-emulsion are frequently generated in a fluid state, with many inconvenience types, including poor stability, irreversible drug/excipient precipitation, high dosage quantities, difficulty handling and transport and limited option for dosage development.

As a possible remedy for these issues, Solid SEDDS (S-SEDDS) was studied. The liquid self-emulsification systems must be powdered to produce different solid-dosage forms (SE capsules, SE tablets, SE pellets, SE beads, and so on). By turning liquid SEDDS into a solid form of dose, the properties of drug release may be preserved. The contents provided by GIT shall be subject to self-emulsification. The benefits of SEDDS are thus coupled with those of a solid dosage form (i.e. increased solubility and bioavailability). Over recent years, the benefits of solid dose as a viable alternative to traditional liquid SEDDS have been examined extensively by using S-SEDDS. Dexibuprofen S-SEDDS, Nimodipine and hydrochlorothiazide are only a few examples. S-SEDDS means solid forms of dosage, which have self-emulsifying characteristics in respect to dose forms. S-SEDDS focuses on the integration into powders and nanoparticles of liquid-semisolid SE components by using various solidification methods.

1.13. Solidification Techniques for Transforming Liquid SEDDS to Solid SEDDS(S-SEDDS) [99-101]

Solid SEDDS is produced via solid carrier adsorbents, spray dries, freezer sealants, melt extruders and liquid/semi-solid SEDDS nanoparticles. SE nanoparticles, drought emulsions and solid dispersions in the many kinds of solid SE dosage are typically processed or put on capsules (i.e., SE capsules). In addition, without solidification excipients SE capsules may also be filled directly with liquid/semisolid SEDDS. SE pellets/tablets, SE microspheres/nanoparticles and SEDDS implants were found as well as solid SE pellets/tablets.

1. Adsorption on solid carriers

Solid carriers employing liquid SE formulations may be adsorbed to free flowing powder. Adsorption is a fundamental procedure which has to be placed and mixed on inert carriers. Before placing it in capsules, it is necessary to crush the resultant powder into tablets or to combine with appropriate excipients. SEDDS may be adsorbed to appropriate high level carriers (up to 70% w/w). Inorganic micro-porosity adsorbs inorganic, colloidal adsorbents of high ranking, polymers or nanoparticles crosslinking Silica, Silicate, Trisilicate of Magnesium, Aluminum Silicate of Magnesium (Neusilin), Calcium silicate (Florite). Self-emulsifying powder is produces using fluid SEDDS adsorption of Neusilin to improve the solubility's of hydrochloride of lercanidipine with poor solubility. Cross-linked polymers enhance environmental drug breakdown. For example, porous silicone dioxide, carbon nanotubes, carbon nanohorns and other adsorbent nanoparticles.

2. Spray drying

The SEDDS fluid is mixed to produce an emulsion o/w by using a suitable solid carrier solution. It then atomizes into a droplet spray in a draining chamber that evaporates the volatile phase, leaking dry particles under regulated temperature and air flow conditions (e.g. emulsion water). These particles may be utilized in the production of tablets or capsules.

3. Freezing techniques

Heat and mass are transported from and to the product during freeze drying or freezing. The freezing of an emulsion of oil-in-water may be possible. Lyophilization is a method of molecular mixing that mixes medicines and transports freeze and sublimate, thereby creating the lyophilized molecular dispersion in the same solvent. It was effectively studied the potential of freeze-drying in solid dispersion production. A low refractive rate and amorphous cryoprotector were discovered to best stabilize the emulsion from oil in water. In the production of freeze-dried tablets, Maltodextrins also are utilized as matrix forming component.

4. Melt granulation

Melt granulation is the powder agglomeration method that uses lipid at low temperatures to melt and/or soften. Melt granulation offers many benefits over traditional wet granulation, as a result of the removal of fluid input and after drying. It is also a possible alternative to the use of solvents. The dissolving rate for glycerides is quicker than previously due of its SE feature as a mix of mono/di/triglycerides and polyethylene glycol ester (PEG). Melt granulations with solid SE were generated utilizing lipid-based excipients such lecithin, partial glycerides and polysorbates. At normal temperature, the lipid excipients must be half-solid.

5. Melt Extrusion/Extrusion spheronization

Melt extrusion is a non-resolvent method that offers (up to 60%) high drug loading and compositional uniformity. Extrusion is a technique used to apply plastic characteristics to a raw material that achieves a consistent, dense output via a die at a regulated temperature, product flow, and pressure. The extruder opening size influences the approximate dimensions of the generated spheroids. Extrusion spheronization is a popular method for the reliable production of large pharmaceutical spheroids (pellets). The sheronizers include a dry combination of active components and excipients for uniform powder, humid massage with a binder, removal into a cable-like extrudate, spheronizing from the extruders to standardized spheroids, drying and scrubbing for the required size and covers distribution.

1.13.1. Advantages of S-SEDDS

- Spontaneous formation
- Ease of manufacture
- Thermodynamic stability and improved solubilization of bioactive materials
- More consistent temporal profiles of drug absorption
- Greater bioavailability
- Less drug needs to be used
- Faster release rates

Medicines suitable in the GI tract for a certain absorption window and resistant to the severe introductive environment. Such techniques may enhance the absorption rate and extent by decreasing the rate of dissolution of lipophilic medicines, creating more repetitive blood time profiles and perhaps lower treatment or drug costs.

1.14. Anthelmintic Therapy [102-106]

Anthelmintics are antifungal worm drugs used to treat parasitic worm infestations. It includes flat worms (e.g., flukes and tapeworms) and circular worms (e.g., nematodes). Based on its anthelmintic prescription, they are essential for tropical and veterinary medications and are a wide spectrum of therapies. Around 2 billion people suffer from parasite worm illnesses, the World Health Organization said. These parasites may damage animals and crops, limit food output and cost money. While parasitic worms are common, anthelmintic drug research in pharmaceutical companies is unfortunate. Helminths may be found all over the place, but more common and fatal illnesses in poor countries. Helminth transmission is all influenced by climate, sanitation, diet and vector exposure.

- Infection: Helminth illness, depending on the type of worm, has been transmitted by egg or larvae, by penetration, by vector meat dough, or by flesh consumption. Worms lengthy lives. Worms long lives.
- Pathogenesis: Most of the infections are asymptomatic and the disease indicates the size, function, and metabolism of the worms, Immune and inflammatory responses may potentially cause pathology. Most people are asymptomatic when they become ill at first. Some people may have stomach pain, diarrhoea and fever if the small intestine of the worms breaks and the intestinal wall. In extreme (and sometimes deadly) circumstances, larvae may enter the heart muscle and brain tissue.
- Host defence: Antibodies and cells mediated responses are required to be inflammatory. Non-specific defence mechanisms decrease their sensitivity. A number of evasive detection methods are used by parasites.
- Diagnosis: Helminth problems are detected by medically, physical examination, faece, and other laboratory tests.
- Treatment: Hands must be frequently washed, bathrooms and kitchens must be cleaned routinely and the food infesting them must be fully cooked. Chlorinated water should be utilized whenever possible. Vermifuges are most often used to kill worms that are very strong anti-worm medications.

Parasite worms depend entirely for survival on their hosts. In order to perpetuate their species, they need to be able to escape from the host body and their progeny (eye or larvae); helminthis eggs or larvae generally do not cause a new host to be infected. They must be able to enter the host body. In the event of oxyurids, it is necessary to return for many hours to prevent parasites from spreading in other parasites before any preventive action may be taken. This crucial step of the helminth life cycle needs to be well understood. A third of the human populations are affected by helminths infections and, in the majority of instances, multiple infections. Helminth infections are common in tropical areas but are afflicted by more than 40 million Americans. In addition, because a broad variety of parasite illnesses may be caused by a large number of domestic animals, these diseases pose a major economic problem for the animal industry.

Helminthiasis is a helminth disease caused by parasites that live in people and the intestines of animals. People with helminthiasis deposit in their faeces worm eggs. These eggs contaminate the soil in places with prevailing or insufficient open defeat. The eggs have a moist floor, and the larvae or eggs are infected with food (red or whip worm) or by the skin (hook worm). Soil helminthiasis is one of the world's most common and neglected tropical diseases, impacting over two billion of the world's poorest populations. It is thought that it takes less than half a year per person to guard against soil-borne helminthiasis. It is estimated that Helminthiasis is 12.5% to 66% of India's population. Helminthiasis affects 50% of the urban population and 68% of the rural population, according to research. Furthermore, using the life years adjusted for handicap the international burden of helminthiasis is evaluated. It is predicted that TB DALY (34.7 million) and malaria (39 million) will be comparable to 39 million DALY years (DALYs) (46.5 million DALYs). Although the number of diseases is small, mortality kills about 5.00 thousand people annually.

The anthelmintic drug Praziquantel is categorized. It works by removing parasites from the body. Parasites are also paralyzed so that they lose hold of the blood artery's walls and are naturally expelled from the body. Because of its large efficacy, minimal toxicities and simple oral administration, PZQ remained the favored therapy for all forms of schistosomiasis in people compared with two other major schistosomiasis medicines: metrifonate and oxamniquine. PZQ was the first anthelmintic to follow the requirements for parasite chemical therapeutic illness in the population of the World Health Organization (WHO). Nearly a million patients were treated with PZQ by 1985. In this respect, the creation of PZQ might be regarded as an example of how tropical diseases have been successfully developed.

The present study aims to formulate and evaluate a stable self-emulsifying drug delivery system (SEDDS) of poorly water-soluble drug Praziquantel to enhance the solubility and oral bioavailability, which provide better with decrease dosing frequency and hence produces better patient compliance.

1.15. Regulatory view

Traditionally, excipients are regarded inert chemicals primarily utilized for manufacturing pharmaceutical formulations as diluents and binders, lubricants, coatings, solvencies and colours (Handbook of Pharmaceutical Excipients). The progress in pharmaceutical research and technology, however, has contributed to make accessible a broad variety of new excipients over the years. However, not all excipients are currently recognised as inert (http://www.fda.gov/cder/guidance/5544fnl.pdf). In the Code of Federal Regulations (CFR), FDA has issued lists of GRAS drugs with broad approvals (USFDA, Title 21, Code of Federal Regulations, Part 182, 184, 186.). Over the years the Agency has kept a list of approved excipients for a commercialized product called the Inactive Ingredients Guide (http://www.fda.gov/cder/drug/iig/default.htm).

This handbook is useful since by administration or dosage the dose level is the maximum for each excipient. For the development of medicinal goods, the industry may utilize GRAS lists and IIG data. When an inactive ingredient is found in a medical product approved for a specific route of administration, and a further study may be necessary when it is next included in a new pharmaceutical product. For example, if a particular resistance in a specific dose shape is allowed to a certain inactive component, the sponsor may deem it acceptable for a related product in a similar way. Prior to usage in non-clinical and clinical trials, the safety of a novel excipient is usually established. The US FDA has issued a guideline paper (http://www.fda.gov/cder/guidance/5544fnl.pdf) for non- clinical safety assessments of novel industrial pharmaceutical excipients. Not only the toxicity data for evaluating whether a possible new excipient is safe, but also the safety assessments of excipients used in general and generic medications are included in this Guide. This Guide paper also discusses the suggested short, medium and long-term pharmaceutical testing methods. More significantly, this guideline stresses the necessity to evaluate risk/benefit of new medical product excipients and to set acceptable and safe excipient limitations. Excipient toxicity may frequently be assessed as well as well planned has been demonstrated. Some excipients may replace specific non-clinical safety data with existing human data. In addition, an excipient recorded in the context of previous humans may not need a complete toxicity assessment battery (http://www.fda.gov/cder/guidance/5544fnl.pdf). Under the conditions relevant to his intended application. As the excipients represent a significant component of the formula and it cannot be evaluated independently from the medical product, the regulatory method is scientifically acceptable. In particular, this applies to lipid excipients, due to their unique physical and chemical characteristics and their very complicated interactions with other components.

2. LITERATURE SURVEY

- **Maria Saifee et al., (2013)** formulated and evaluated Solid Self- Emulsifying Drug Delivery System (SEDDS) of glibenclamide. The objective of this investigation was to establish a strong self-emulsifying Aerosil 200 system to increase the dissolution rate of glibenclamide models (GBM). Capmul MCM C8TM, Cremophor RH 40 and Transcutol were respectively utilized for the production of SEDDS as oil, surfactant and co-surfactant. In the microemulsion region of oil and water a pseudo-ternary phase diagram was discovered to produce a stable SEDDS (1:1, 2:1 and 3:1). SEDDS preparation evaluated turbidity, globule dimensions and zeta potential, viscosity evaluation and % transmittance. Using the solid carrier adsorption technique Aerosil 200, S-SEDDS was developed. S-SEDDS was used to generate all flow features, pharmaceutical drug content, FTIR, SEM, DSC and the study of *in vitro* dissolution. The liquid SEDDS was used to perform all experiments. The globule size was measured as 142.8 nm and polydispersity index to 0.396.

- **Fariba Khan et al., (2012)** have carried out a comprehensive bioavailability research for Atorvastatin Self-Emulsifying Drug Delivery Systems. The study was intended to develop and characterize a self-emulsifying drug delivery system (SEDDS), which is deficient in water solubility owing to a large drug load on atorvastatin for improved oral dispersion. The solubility of atorvastatin in oils, surfactants and cosurfactants has been evaluated via research. The water titration technique was employed and formulations were based on pseudoternary diagrams of phases, depending on optimum excipient combinations. The combination of oleic acid, Tween 80 and polyethylene glycol 400 produced significant (10% w/w) medications of excellent resolution.

- **Hong JY. et al., (2006)** have created novel auto-emulsifying formulations of itraconazole by improving dissolution and oral absorption. The surfactants and oil with the highest solubility in Itraconazole are chosen for transcutol, pluronic L64 and tocopherol acetate. Itraconazole solubility is significantly improved by the use of hydrochloric acid. During the incubation process of 120 minutes the itraconazole emulsion droplet was constantly maintained, simulating stomach pH 1.2 and intestinal fluid (pH 6.8). In the ddissolution mmedium in SEDDS, the Itraconazole was dissolved very rapidly; in the incubation period 120 minutes, depending on the dissolving media, Sporanox exhibited various dissolving patterns. Following SEDDS, the fasting and feeding group were compared to itraconazole, AUC (0 —>24h) and Maximal itraconazole plasma (Cmax) after oral Sporanox.

- **Saritha Damineni et al., (2014)** has developed and evaluated an independent ibuprofen emulsification medication delivery procedure (SEDDS). For oil, surfactant and co-surfactant, Labrafac, Tween 80 and PEG 200 were chosen. For design and screen composition, the results of phase diagrams and the characteristics of the resultant microemulsions were utilized. SEDDS scans were performed to assess the droplet size, zeta potential, polydispersibility index, viscosity, refractive index, % transmittance, drug content and *in vitro* dissolution profile. The SEDDS formulations showed an excellence in the continuous stabilization, creaming or breaking, micrometer-sized globules and transparent emulsions generated rapidly. Over 90% of the medication was administered in all formulations in 30 minutes.

- **Sharmin Nipun Tanzina et al., (2014)** used Gliclazide SEDDS methods *in vitro*, ex vivo and *in vivo*. Oils and surfactant solubilizers have been employed to filter out them. The components under review showed excellent solubilizing effects for Transcutol HP and Tween-80. Both components were mixed to produce SEDDS Gliclazide in different quantities. The SEDDS formula was simple and clear. The droplet size emulsion was calculated using Malvern's laser diffraction technology. The lowest mean transcutol HP/Tween-80 droplet size was 1:1 in formulation F1 (50.959 μm). *In vitro* drug release of F1 was higher than in other formulations (99% within 20 minutes). An extra chicken intestinal bag was provided for the ex-vivo SEDDS permeability profile. The delivery of medical goods was the most important element of Formulation F1. The performance of *in vivo* SEDDS in albino mice has been assessed using Plasma Glucose.

- **Fahim Tamzeedul Karim et al., (2012)** have been developed and manufactured by Simvastatin SEDDS. According to their water solubility, oils and surfactants were assessed. For all solvents, Capryol 90 offers the finest solutions. Dissolved to 105 mg/ml of Simvastatin. Similarly, 117 mg/ml were considerably soluble for Tween-80. Both excipients produced the Simvastatin SEDDS. Colour, clarity and sedimentation were the first test. The SEDDS formula was simple and clear. F2 comprising Capryol 90 and Tween-80 combinations generated and discharged at least 0.074 mm of microemulsion and more than any other medications; (102% within 20 min.). The SEDDS formula was ex vivo using a guinea pig intestinal bag. There was a significantly greater volume of medicines supplied by F2 than pure medication. In the SEDDS *in vivo* research albino mice plasma cholesterol was assessed using pharmacodynamic assessment.

- **Cui S. X. et al., (2009)** prepared a SMEDDS including 15% oils, 50% Surfactants, and 35% cosurfactants, for improved vinpocetine bioavailability. SE formula release rates were much greater than tablets. Vinpocetine SMEDDS has an oral bioavailability 1.72 times higher than the regular tablets. Vinpocetine SMEDDS absorption has improved significantly.

- **Elnaggar Y. S. et al., (2009)** told Tamoxifen citrate is an anti-estrogenic chemistry. The chemical used to treat peroral breast cancer is Tamoxifen citrate. It has issues such as water solution, intestinal degradation and hepatic degradation. For optimal component combinations, such solubility tests, preliminary screening was carried out. Then the excipients were selected by using ternary phase diagrams. In order to enhance its robust dilution, measurements of globule size, surface morphology and drug release, these three formulations of SNEDDS Tamoxifen were further evaluated. Dilutions and different dilution levels were not a problem for an system. With 80°C cloud point, the system measured at 150 nm globule size. On a TEM scan, spherical particles emerged. In contrast to drug suspension, the release of medications from the chosen SNEDDS was high. The findings indicate that if administered orally, the improved SNEDDS system may boost the value of the poorly soluble tamoxifen medication.

- **Balakrishnan P. et al., (2009)** developed a solid SE system to increase bioavailability dexibuprofen. The liquid SE System combines drugs with excipients (Capryol 90, Labrasol & Labrafil). The emulsions of the fluid and the solid SE system did not vary from the particle size. The initial medicinal plasma concentrations of the solid-SE system in comparisons between solid-SE and medicinal powder were considerably greater than those of the drug powder. The solid SE system AUC and Cmax have been improved compared to medications. This showed solid SEDDS enhanced bioavailability of dexibuprofen.

- **N. Zhang et al., (2011)** created the super SMEDDS Carbamazepine, compared with an *in-vitro* dissolution and distribution of particle size in a trade behavioral tablet and related biological accessible dogs. The size of the SMEDDS was 33.7 nm and with an AUC five times the size of the commercial tablets, the release rate was considerably higher. The result has been an efficient method of increasing Carbamazepine absorption by Carbamazepine S-SMEDDS.

- **J. Patel et al., (2011)** developed SNEDDS to improve telmisartan bioavailability. The oil phase was chosen after a solubility investigation. For emulsifying oil, surfactants and co-surfactants have been chosen. On the basis of a ternary phase diagram the SE area was estimated. All SNEDDS evaluations were performed via % transmittance, globule size and zeta potential, viscosity, drug content, emulsification study and dilution tests. Optimized SNEDDS of telmisartan consisted of 20 mg Telmisartan, 43.33% Tween 20, 21.67% Carbitol and 32% of Acrysol EL 135. It gave complete drug release in 15 min & 7.5 folds bioavailability improvement compared to drug. It was found that SNEDDS improved dissolution of telmisartan and also enhanced its oral bioavailability.

- **A. Chudasama et al., (2011)** has created a SEDDS system for lipid nevirapine to target the most identified lymphocytes of HIV-1. Based on their solubility and ternary phase diagrams, the nevirapine SEDDS components were chosen. The optimized formulation included Caprylic acid (8.56%), soluphor P (74.5%) and transcutol P co-surfactant. (16.93%). The spherical globules were smaller than 200 nm in diameter. *In vitro* diffusion exhibited 99.18 ⊥ 2.85% nevirapine release from SEDDS as compared to 65.14 + 2.98% release from the marketed formulation. Ex-vivo intestinal permeability was also found to be higher from SEDDS than marketed suspension.

- **S. Gupta et al., (2011)** has been produced Adefovir dipivoxil SNEDDS by due to their low permeability, pH based solubility and bioavailability. By increased intestinal penetration and lower pH sensitivity, the bioavailability of the medication is improved. Excipients were chosen after a preliminary screening. The nano-emulsifying zone has been created by using phase diagrams. By using cryoprotectant D-mannitol in the optimized system was transformed into solid SNEDDS. It described as the robust system. In the liquid system, the globule size were 110±10 nm and the solid system showed 150±16 nm. The new formulation of the cloud point is between 80-85°C. Spherical globules were found in the SEM and TEM nanoemulsion study. Medicines in solid systems have also been evaluated by using DSC and XRD. In pH globular size or temperature changes, no significant modifications were observed. *In-vitro* as well as ex-vivo release from system were significantly higher compared to plain drug suspension. Thus, solid SNEDDS proven to be instrumental to decrease the pH effect and to enhance drug release. So, they proved potential for improvement of bioavailability and efficacy of drug.

- **N. Parmar et al., (2011)** Enhanced oral bioavailability of lercanidipine SNEDDS. Excipients were chosen according to their solubility. It is then generated a ternary phase diagram. Dispersibility experiments and thermodynamic investigations were followed by several formulations. Co-surfactants have been studied in the nano-emulsification zone. Viscosity measurements, % transmittance, SE time and droplet size were characteristic of this substance. Optimized SNEDDS included 45% Cremophore EL, 13.5% Capryol 90, 1.5% Transcutol HP and 10% Corn Oil. Tablets and medications were extremely large on the market and with various pH buffers. The droplet size in formulations was 20.01 nm. The filled HGC undergone for various temperature and humidity testing for three months, then it remained unaltered. LER method to increase the use of medications has proven SNEDDS to be successful.

- **A. Meena et al., (2012)** Solubility and dissolution of albendazole (ABZ) was successfully enhanced for the purposes of increasing systemic exposure. Based on surfactants and oils, SEDDS was created. The SEDDS receptor increases solubility and systemic exposure, by examining emulsifying characteristics, droplet diameters, dissolution and other factors, compared to lipophilic anthelmintic, pharmaceuticals such as ABZ.

- **Bhagwat D. A. et al., (2012)** were developed telmisartan SMEDDS. Oleic acid, PEG 400 and Tween 80 were used as excipients. The microemulsion area was shown in a ternary phase diagram. For emulsification investigations, SE systems were described. In the solid system Neusilin US2 was added and analyzed for flow properties, FTIR, DSC, SEM and dissolution study. At 30.2 nm globule size , 0.116 PDI and -5.8 mV of zeta potential, the liquid solution was thermodynamically stable. The solid system with 32.4 nm globule size, 0.219 PDI and − 6.32 mV zeta potential exhibited an efficient flow and good reconstitution. The method proposed enhanced the dissolving rate of telmisartan as compared to a dissolution experiment. Neusilin US2 has shown to be an adsorption carrier to produce solid, poorly soluble SMEDDS for telmisartan.

- **U. Goyal et al. (2012)**, have checked self-emulsification efficiency of lovastatin via resolution of the issue of oral bioavailability by administration of solution. Capryol 90 (20%), Cremophore RH40 (40%) and transcutol P co-surfactants were found to offer optimal components using saturated solvency tests, an emulsifying capacity and ternary stage diagrams (40%). The droplet size, zeta potential, emulsification time, rheological tests and TEM were all investigated for SMEDDS. The optimized formulation revealed a 94% drug release rate much greater than the pure medicine solution. *In vivo* the levels of cholesterol in comparison to pure lovastatin were considerably lower.

- **N. Choudhary et al., (2014)** explores SEDDS to improve the bioavailability of Eprosartan. For Oil Labrafac WL following saturation solubility testing, the surfactants Tween 80 and Capryol 90 have been chosen. Self-emulsifying area ternary phase diagrams have been utilized. Characterization experiments were conducted to increase the formulation, including the % transmittance, self emulsification time, dilution studies, thermodynamic studies and blood measurement. An impact on the size of globules was examined with the excipient concentration. A substantial 98.3% drug release was generated by the adjusted formula. The oral bioavailability and absorption of Eprosartan from SEDDS found to be enhanced compared to aqueous suspension *in vivo*.

- **Venkatesh G. et al., (2010)** is prepared SMEDDS to improve the buparvaquone (BPQ), solubility and bioavailability. A number of characterization tests have been conducted including emulsification time and droplet sizes. Dissolution and pharmacokinetic testing have been carried out to optimize the product. For Buparvaquone, the SMEDDS was optimal at 1.78%, 9.82% for Capryol 90, 70.72% for Cremophore EL and 17.68% for Labrasol The overall release rate for both SGF-SIF drugs in 90 minutes was 100%. The bioavailability of Buparvaquone is 40.10%. SMEDDS enhances the absorption of buparvaquone and is orally appropriate.

- **Varinkova et al., (2015)** This research focuses on the development and testing of improved *in vitro* testing and evaluation of the differences in liquids and alumino metasilicate (NeusilinUS2) systems (polyethylene glycol 400 solution of rosuvastatin). Two alternative techniques were used to build the final tablet by using granules. The drug solution was easily manufactured and sprayed on a fluidized bed. The results show that the amount of the liquid phase of the conveyor material leads to durability, decay, dissolution and durability. Using spray drying technique enhances the mixing flow characteristics, boosts hardness, minimizes crushing strength and increases dose consistency.

- **Amrutkar et al., (2014)** The SNEDDS system is ready to improve rosuvastatin calcium solubility and bioavailability. The three phase diagram was based on the calcium solubility assessment for the improvement of rosuvastatin systems. The emulsification time, dispersion studies, average pellet volume and PDI have been examined. There are smaller than 100 nm of system optimum cell size and this may be an acceptable nanometer. The mean cell size was found to be 88.02 nm for SNEDDS of F2 formulation (20 % Capmul MCM and 40% PEG 200). Research in the laboratory on the release of drugs has shown a substantial increase in dissociation from F2 SNEDDS.

- **Shinde et al., (2014)** The biological oral dosage is compared with one of the lovastatin nanoparticles in white rabbits. Plasma formulation concentration has been used to establish pharmacological parameters like AUC, Cmax, Tmax, t1/2, MRI and Kel. Random divisions into three groups, comprising Standards-I, Standards-II and testing, with six animals in each category. Pure Lovastatin has been prepared and marketed by default with lovastatin. Nanoparticles loaded with lovastatin were suspended for the test group. The bioavailability of relative bioavailability is substantially improved in comparison with traditional tablets (1.5 times).

- **Qureshi et al., (2015)** The statistical data for the self-emulsifying drug system were created and enhanced by (SMEDDS). On dry liquid-filled tablets, the SMEDDS was directly sprayed on magnesium aluminium metasilicate. The co-ordinated version of SMEDDS shows that the SMEDDS formula's lovastatin profile is much higher than that of lovastatin alone. Then the changed form was put in the magnesium powder and immediately adsorbed to disc building. They also consider the potential of using magnesium aluminometasilicate to advantage hyperbolic, healthy dietary rabbits. SMEDDS fluid was also used to deliver the rabbits, which was proven to work with SMEDDS solid, magnesium and aluminium.

- **Krupa et al., (2014)** fluid layer coating Ibuprofen SEDDS produces permeable granules using a method of extrusion, magnesium aluminometasilicate. Examine if the granules can be utilized in solid SEDDS fluid converting (S-SEDDS). For the formation of extrusion granules Neusilin, SG2, US2 and NS2N are utilized with MCC (Microcrystalline Cellulose). Higher porosity and mechanical resistance were observed in the Neusilin SG2 pellets. The technique for covering fluid beds with liquid ibuprofen SEDDS has been shown. This research shows that over 80% ibuprofen has been dissolved in weight in the phosphate buffer pH 6.8 by the combination of 70% Neusilin SG2 after 30 minutes.

- **Rokade et al., (2014)** The distribution method for improving the solubility and oral bio-availability of solid calcium rosuvastatin capsules was developed and tested using the smallest quantity of surface agents. Rosuvastatin has been assessed by using the optical spectrum technique in different oils, surfactants and surfactants. Cremophore EL and propylene glycol were chosen on the basis of solubility testing, as an oil, surfactant and cosurfactant. It was then adsorbed to create solid, physical SMEDDS and SMEDDS fluid was developed. In addition to the commercial formulations, the dosage of S-SEDDS rosuvastatin was released that may replace the low-solutions medication in water.

4. AIM &OBJECTIVES

AIM

The aim of study was to "Formulation and Optimization of Self Emulsifying Drug Delivery System for Effective Anthelmintic Therapy"

OBJECTIVES

The main objective of this study is to improve the solubility of the medicine by utilizing self-emulsifying drug delivery system and to create flexible solid oral dose for pediatric patients. This overall goal is split into the following support objectives;

1. To formulate liquid self-emulsifying drug delivery system containing praziquantel as a drug with suitable oil, surfactant and co-surfactant.
2. To characterize the prepared formulations.
3. To carry out anthelmintic study from optimized liquid SEDDS formulation.
4. To perform solidification of liquid SEDDS into a solid SEDDS by physical adsorption onto inert solid material.
5. To formulate and evaluate solid self-emulsifying drug delivery system.
6. To compare the dissolution profile of optimized tablet formulation with that of marketed product.
7. To formulate taste masked oral formulations.
8. To carry out *in vivo* pharmacokinetic study from optimized tablet formulation.
9. To evaluate the stability study of P-L-SEDDS and P-S-SEDDS.

5. PLAN OF WORK

- Literature survey
- Selection and procurement of drug and excipients
- Preformulation study
- Experimental design and work
    - ✓ Screening of various oils, surfactants and co-surfactants for maximum solubilization of drug.
    - ✓ Construction of Pseudo-ternary phase diagrams.
    - ✓ Formulation of liquid self emulsifying drug delivery system by using Central composite design.
    - ✓ Characterization of developed formulation.
        - Visual observation
        - Emulsification time
        - Globule size analysis
        - Determination of Zeta potential
        - Microscopic evaluation
        - Effect of surfactant concentration
        - Effect of cosurfactant concentration
        - *In vitro* drug release
        - Anthelmintic activity
- To assess the stability study of optimized Liquid SEDDS formulation.
- Conversion of liquid SEDDS to solid SEDDS.
- *IN-VITRO* evaluation of developed solid self-emulsifying drug delivery system.
- To formulate taste masked oral formulation.
- *IN-VIVO* studies of optimized S-SEDDS formulation.

6. DRUG AND EXCIPIENTS PROFILE

DRUG PROFILE [107-109]

Table 2. Physicochemical properties of Praziquantel

Name	Praziquantel
Description	White or almost white crystalline powder.
Pharmacopoieal specification	Official in IP,USP, BP & European Pharmacopoeia
Molecular formula	C19H24N2O2
Structure	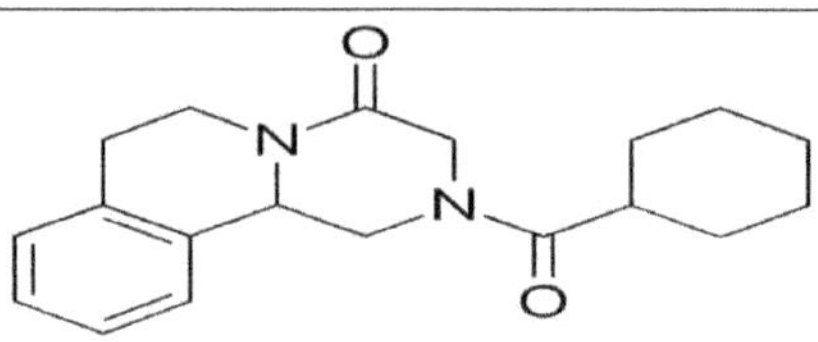
IUPAC Name	2-(cyclohexylcarbonyl)-1,2,3,6,7,11b-hexahydro-4H-pyrazino[2,1-a] isoquinolin-4-one.
Molecular weight	312.4 g/mol.
Melting Point	136°C–141°C
Log P	2.42
PKa	19.38
Half-life	0.8-1.5 hr.
Solubility	1. Very slightly soluble in water. 2. Soluble in methanol, ethanol, chloroform and dimethylsulfoxide
Class	Anthelmintics
Dose	20 mg/kg
Mechanism of Action	Praziquantel acts by inducing severe muscular spasms and paralysis in the worm. This paralysis is supported by a fast influx of Ca^{2+} inside the schistosome and is probably caused. Morphological changes are another early impact. While it is beneficial against schistosomes, it gradually loses its effectivity till after 3-4 weeks.

Pharmacokinetics **1. Absorption**	80% of the given PZQ dosage is absorbed after oral administration and susceptible to a first pass effect.
2. Distribution	The volume of distribution is around 8000 L. & PZQ is between 80-85% bound to plasma proteins.
3. Metabolism	The cytochrome P450 enzyme is quickly metabolized to generate the PZQ medication following oral administration of Biltricide.
4. Excretion	Approximately 80% of the oral dosage of Biltricide is excreted in the kidneys, virtually entirely in the form of PZQ metabolites (more than 99%).
Pharmacodynamics	The PZQ medication reduces the permeability of the cell membrane of schistosome species. The schistosome tegument is likewise vacuolized and disintegrated. Side effects include reduction of glucose absorption, decreased glycogen and stimulation of lactate release.
Indication	For the treatment of all schistosoma species infections.
Side effects	➢ Dizziness ➢ Headache ➢ Abdominal pain ➢ Nausea

EXCIPIENTS PROFILE

1. **Capmul MCM [110]**

Table 3. Physicochemical properties of Capmul MCM

Synonyms	Glycerol Monocaprylate, Glyceryl Mono- & Dicaprylate, Medium Chain Mono-& Diglycerides.
Chemical name	Monoglyceride of capylic acid
CAS Registry Number	26402-26-2
Empirical Formula	C11H22O4
Molecular weight	218.29 g/mol

Physical state at 20⁰ C	Liquid
Melting point	48°C
Appearance	Colorless to yellow liquid
Odor	Fatty odor
Structural formula	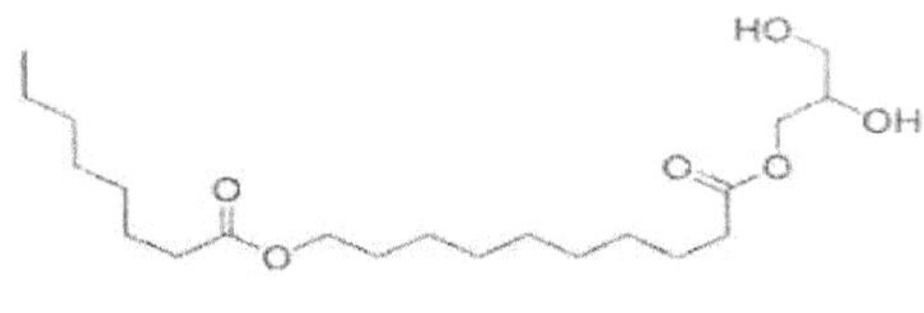
HLB Value	5 – 6
Solubility	It is miscible with chloroform, diethyl ether, ethanol and glacial acetic acid and methanol; it is easily soluble in ethanol (95%) and petroleum ether, is virtually insoluble in water and unless combined with another vegetable oil miscible with water or alcohol, is basically insoluble in mineral oil.
Incompatibility	It is incompatible with strong oxidizing agents.
Applications	➢ Capmul MCM is most preferably used in preparation of emulsion because it acts as a solubilizer for poorly soluble compounds or as a suspension medium to facilitate absorption and improve bioavailability. ➢ Capmul MCM is an emulsifier or co-emulsifier in preparation of stable self-emulsifying lipid-based microemulsions.

2. Cremophor RH 40 [111]

Table 4. Physicochemical properties of Cremophor RH 40

Synonym	Polyoxyl 40 hydrogenated castor oil
CAS Registry Number	61788-85-0 617
Empirical Formula	$C_{68}H_{122}O_{15}$

Molecular weight	1119.6 g/mol
Appearance	White to pale yellow oily liquid
Odor	Odorless
Structural formula	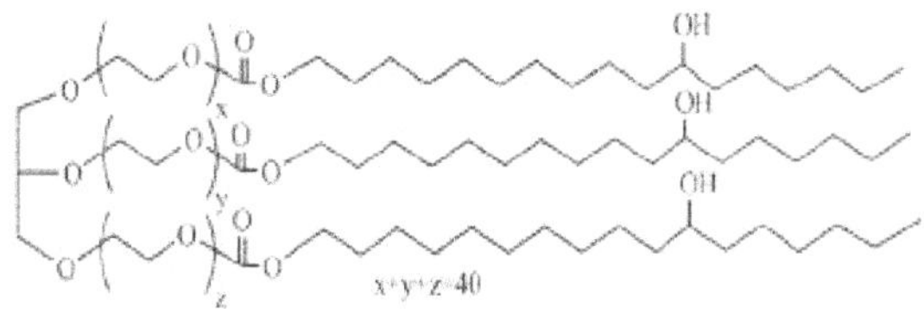
HLB Value	14–16
Solubility	➢ It is soluble in many organic solvents. ➢ It is miscible with oleic and stearic acids, dodecyl and octa-decyl alcohols, castor oil and a number of lipid-soluble substances.
Applications	➢ Cremophore RH 40 is employed in water solubilization of aquatic insoluble active compounds, vitamins and essential oils, as well as water-alcohol combinations. ➢ Also employed as an emulsifying agent is the Cremophore RH 40.

3. Polyethylene Glycol 400 [112]

Table 5. Physicochemical properties of Polyethylene Glycol 400

Synonyms	Carbowax; Carbowax Sentry; Lipoxol; Lutrol E; macrogola; PEG; Pluriol E and polyoxyethylene glycol.
Chemical name	α-Hydro-ω-hydroxypoly (oxy-1,2-ethanediyl)
CAS Registry Number	25322-68-3
Empirical Formula	HOCH2(CH2OCH2)8.7CH2OH
Molecular weight	380-420 g/mol
Colour and Physical form at 25 ° C	Colorless liquid
Melting point	4-8°C

Odor	Characteristic
Structural formula	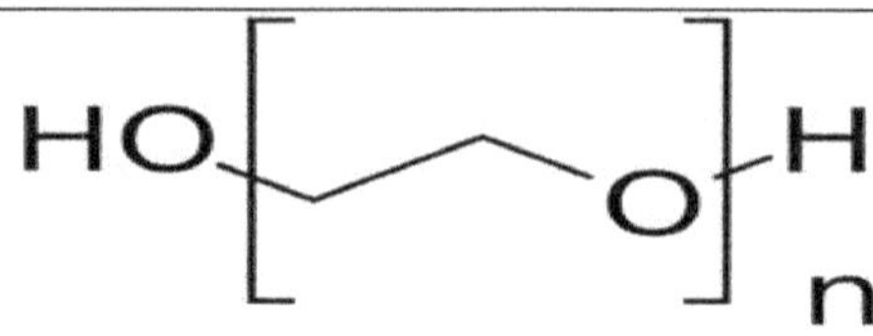
HLB Value	16
Solubility	Liquid polyethylene glycols are soluble in water, acetone, alcohols, benzene, glycerin, and glycols.
Incompatibility	Penicillin, bicitracin, iodine, potassium iodides, sorbitol, tannic acid, bismuth salts are not compatible with glycols. Glycols with polyethylene, backlite and celluloids are also not appropriate.
Applications	➢ A few applications for polyethylene glycols include topical, oral, parenteral, ophthalmic and rectal administration. ➢ Liquid PEG are used widely in lipid-based medicaments such as solid dispersion and self-emulsifying mixtures because they are water miscible co-solvents with good solvent properties for water-soluble drugs.

4. Aerosil 200 [113,114]

Table 6. Physicochemical properties of Aerosil 200

Synonyms	Aerosil; Aeropearl 300 pharma; Cab-O-Sil; Cab-O-SilM-5P; colloidal silica; fumed silica; fumed silicon dioxide and hoch disperses silicum dioxide.
Chemical name	Silica
CAS Registry Number	7631-86-9
Empirical Formula	SiO2
Molecular weight	60.08 g/mol
Colour and Physical form at 25 ° C	Bluish-white amorphous powder
Melting point	1600°C

Odor	Odorless
Solubility	It is practically insoluble in water, organic solvents and acids, except hydrofluoric acid; and soluble in hot solutions of alkali hydroxide. It produces a colloidal dispersion with water. For Aerosil, solubility in water is 150 mg/L at 258°C (pH 7).
Incompatibility	Incompatible with diethylstilbestrol preparations.
Functional Category	➢ Adsorbent; anti caking agent; emulsion stabilizer; glidant; suspending agent; tablet disintegrant; thermal stabilizer; viscosity-increasing agent; Carrier for liquid and pasty (active) ingredients, Converts liquid and pasty substances into free-flowing powders.

5. Neusilin US2 [115,116]

Table 7. Physicochemical properties of Neusilin US2

Synonyms	Aluminii magnesii silicas; aluminosilicic acid; magnesium aluminum silicate
Chemical name	Magnesium aluminometasilicate
CAS Registry Number	12511-31-8
Empirical Formula	Al2O3.MgO. 7SiO2.xH2O
Chemical Structure	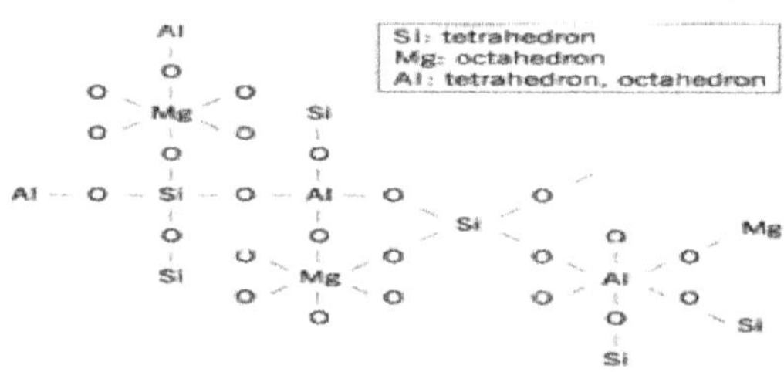
Molecular weight	143.36 g/mol
Appearance	White amorphous powder or granule
Solubility	Practically insoluble in water and ethanol.

Uses	➢ Neusilin US2® is used as a solid dose diluent. ➢ Used as a binder to improve the durability and as a support for disintegration in the manufacture of tablets. ➢ Used as a liquid solidifying agent, Active Pharmaceutical Ingredients (API) / Used to stabilize delicates (stabilizing of unstable pharmaceutical agent / prepare for moisture). ➢ Used as both a compounding and dispersion aid. ➢ Used as an adsorbent.

6. Doshion P-544 DS [117]

Table 8. Physicochemical properties of Doshion P-544 DS

Chemical name	Methacrylic co-Polymer with divinyl benzene
Chemical Structure	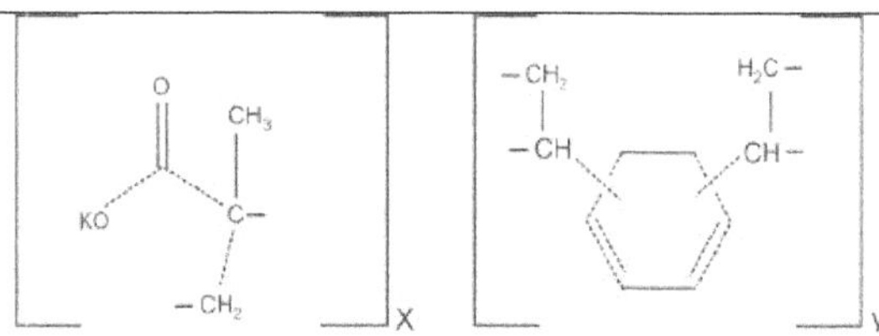
Appearance	White to off-white Powder
Uses	➢ Super disintegration ➢ Dissolution improvement
Advantages	➢ Super rapid Disintegration ➢ Swell rapidly & wicks water by capillary action ➢ Direct compressible grade Elimination of lump formation ➢ Compatibility with other therapeutic agents ➢ Imparts excellent strength to the tablet ➢ Eliminate the sticking to the dyes and punch

7. Croscarmellose sodium [118]

Table 9. Physicochemical properties of Croscarmellose sodium

Synonyms	Croscarmellose, Carboxymethyl cellulose, carboxymethyl ether Cellulose
Chemical name	Cellulose, Carboxy methyl ether, Sodium salt cross linked
Molecular Formula	$C_8H_{16}O_8$
Chemical Structure	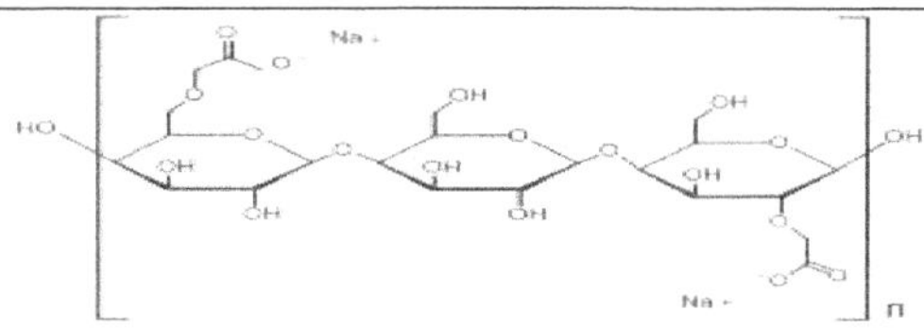
Molecular weight	240.21 g/mol
Description	It as an odourless, white or greyish white powder.
Applications	Used as Disintegrant in Capsules, Tablet and Granule Formulations.
Storage	Stored in Well Closed Container at Cool and Dry Place as Croscarmellose Sodium is Hygroscopic by Nature.

8. Sodium Starch Glycolate [118]

Table 10. Physicochemical properties of Sodium Starch Glycolate

Synonyms	Sodium salt; Carboxy methyl amylum natricum; Explosol; Explotab; Glycols; Primogel; starch carboxy methyl ether; sodium salt; Tablo; Vivastar P.
Chemical name	Sodium carboxy methyl starch
Molecular Formula	C2H4O3·xNa·x
Chemical Structure	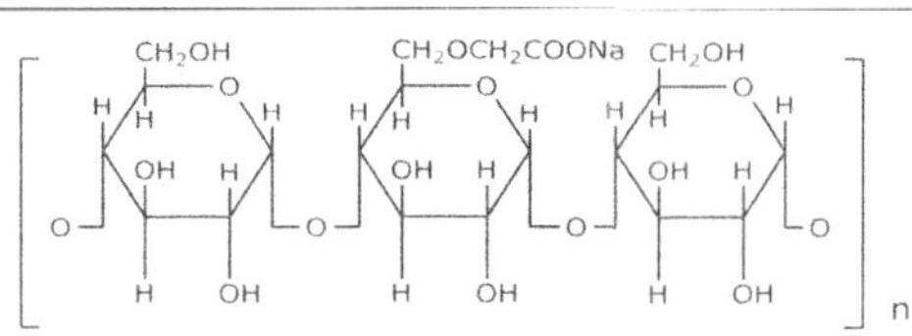

Molecular weight	290.243 g/mol
Appearance	White or almost white, very fine, hygroscopic powder
Applications	➢ Sodium starch glycolate is often used to disintegrate oral pharmaceutical preparations into capsules and tablets. ➢ It is commonly used by either direct or wet-granulation techniques in the manufacture of tablets.
Storage	It should be stored in a container properly closed.

9. Polyplasdone XL-10 [118]

Table 11. Physicochemical properties of Polyplasdone XL-10

Synonyms	Crospovidonum; Crospopharm; crosslinked povidone; E1202;Kollidon CL; Kollidon CL-M; Crospovidone; polyvinylpolypyrrolidone; PVPP; 1-vinyl-2-pyrrolidinone homopolymer
Chemical name	1-Ethenyl-2-pyrrolidinone homopolymer
Chemical Structure	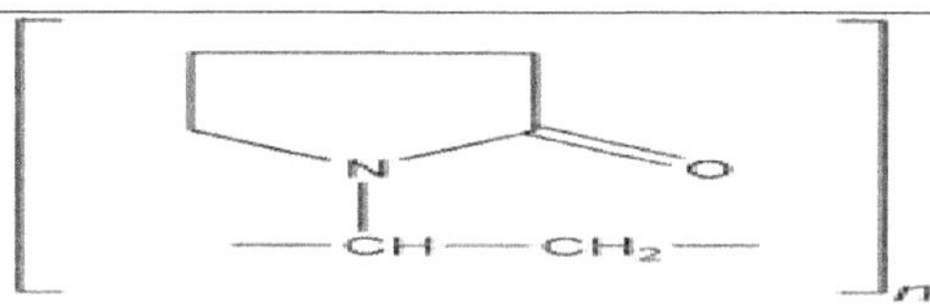
Description	It is a white to creamy-white, finely divided, free flowing, practically tasteless, odourless or nearly odourless, hygroscopic powder.
Advantages	➢ Combines multiple mechanisms to achieve disintegration at low use levels (2-5 wt %) ➢ Swells without forming gels that can slow tablet disintegration or dissolution ➢ Provides rapid disintegration in wet and dry granulations and direct compression tablet processes. It can be added intra- or extra- granularly ➢ Increases tablet breaking force and reduces friability ➢ Enhances the dissolution of poorly soluble drugs.

10. Microcrystalline Cellulose [118]

Table 12. Physicochemical properties of Microcrystalline Cellulose

Synonyms	Avicel PH, Celex, Celphere, Crystalline cellulose, Emcocel, Fibrocel, Pharmacel
Chemical name	Cellulose
Chemical Structure	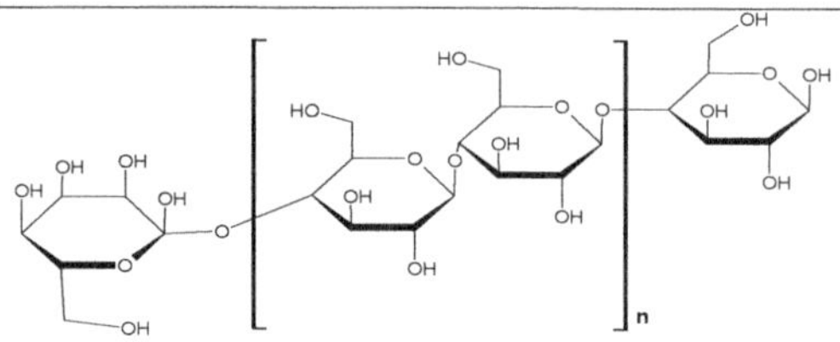
Empirical Formula	$(C_6H_{10}O_5)_n$
Molecular Weight	Approx. 36000
Applications	➢ Microcrystalline cellulose is used as a binder, disintegrating and filler in granulating and tablet preparations as well as in direct compression tablet preparations. ➢ Microcrystalline cellulose is used in a ratio of 20-90% as a tablet binder/diluent and in a ratio of 5-15% as a tablet disintegrant.
Storage	The bulk material should be stored in a cold, dry area in a well-closed container.

11. Povidone [118]

Table 13. Physicochemical properties of Povidone

Synonyms	1-Ethenyl-2-pyrrolidinone polymers 1-ethenylpyrrolidin-2-one 1-Vinyl-2-pyrrolidinone
IUPAC Name	1-ethenylpyrrolidin-2-one
Chemical Structure	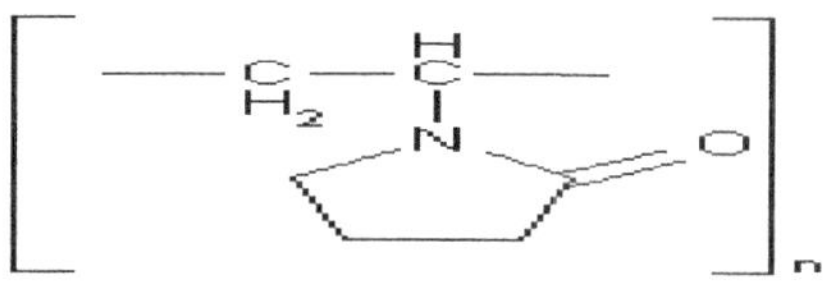
Empirical Formula	C6H9NO (isomer)
Molecular Weight	2500–3,000,000
Applications	➢ Povidone is used in a variety of pharmaceutical formulations, it is primarily used in solid-dosage forms. ➢ In tableting, povidone solutions are used as binders in wet-granulation processes. ➢ Povidone is also added to powder blends in the dry form and granulated in situ by the addition of water, alcohol, or hydroalcoholic solutions. ➢ Povidone is used as a solubilizer in oral and parenteral formulations, and has been shown to enhance dissolution of poorly soluble drugs from solid-dosage forms. ➢ Povidone solutions may also be used as coating agents or as binders when coating active pharmaceutical ingredients on a support such as sugar beads. ➢ Povidone is additionally used as a suspending, stabilizing, or viscosity-increasing agent in a number of topical and oral suspensions and solutions. ➢ The solubility of a number of poorly soluble active drugs may be increased by mixing with povidone.

12. Mannitol [118]

Table 14. Physicochemical properties of Mannitol

Synonyms	Cordycepic acid, Emprove, manna sugar; D-mannite, mannite, mannitolum, Mannogem, Pearlitol
Chemical name	D-Mannitol
Chemical Structure	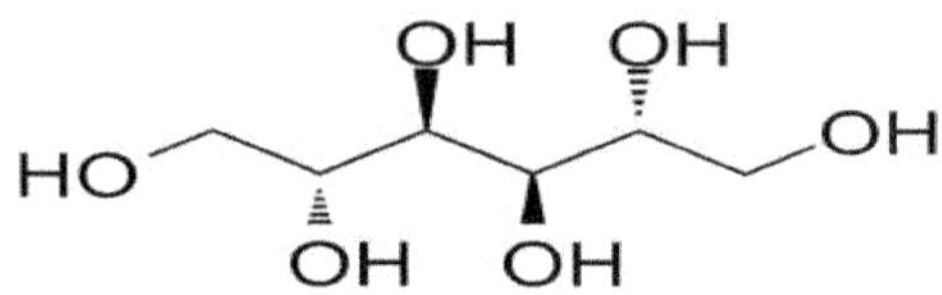
Empirical Formula	$C_6H_{14}O_6$
Molecular Weight	182.17 g/mol
Applications	➢ Mannitol is a polyol or alditol present in various plants and generated by a range of microorganisms. ➢ Mannitol is being utilized for its positive physiological benefits as a functional sweetener in the food sector. ➢ Towards the potential benefits of Mannitol are also uses in the pharmaceutical, chemical and medical sectors. Towards extraction, chemical synthesis, or fermentation, all mannitol may be employed. For a variety of causes, different mutants were produced. In our research, we focused on current advances in the usage of mannitol and the biotechnological production of mannitol.

13. Magnesium Stearate [118]

Table 15. Physicochemical properties of Magnesium Stearate

Synonyms	Dibasic magnesium stearate; magnesium distearate; magnesiistearas; magnesium octadecanoate; octadecanoic acid, magnesium salt; stearic acid, magnesium salt.
Chemical name	Octadecanoic acid magnesium salt
Chemical Structure	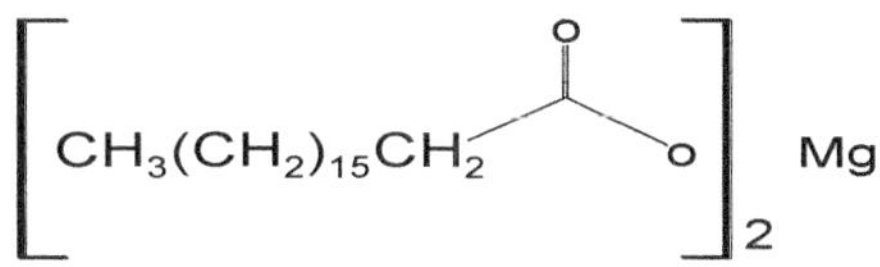
Empirical Formula	$C_{36}H_{70}MgO_4$
Molecular Weight	591.24
Applications	➢ Magnesium stearate is widely used in cosmetics, foods, and pharmaceutical formulations. ➢ It is primarily used as a lubricant in capsule and tablet manufacture at concentrations between 0.25% and 5.0% w/w. ➢ It is also used in barrier creams.

7. MATERIALS AND METHODS

List of Materials

Table 16. List of materials used in present work

Sr. No.	Drug and excipients	Supplier
1	Praziquantel	Microlab Pvt. Ltd., Goa
2	Capmul MCM C8	Abitech Corporation, U.S.A
3	Capryol 90	Gattefosse Limited, France
4	Oleic acid	Pure Chem Laboratory, Pune
5	Arachis oil	Pure Chem Laboratory, Pune
6	Captex 300	Abitech Corporation, U.S.A
7	Castor oil	Pure Chem Laboratory, Pune
8	PEG 400	Pure Chem Laboratory, Pune
9	Castor oil	Pure Chem Laboratory, Pune
10	Soyabean oil	Pure Chem Laboratory, Pune
11	Isopropyl Myristate	Mohini Organics, Mumbai
12	Labrafil	Gattefosse Limited, France
13	Olive oil	Pure Chem Laboratory, Pune
14	Almond oil	Pure Chem Laboratory, Pune
15	Cremophor RH 40	BASF, Mumbai
16	Tween 80	S.D. Fine Chem. Ltd., Mumbai
17	Tween 20	S.D. Fine Chem. Ltd., Mumbai
18	Span 20	S.D. Fine Chem. Ltd., Mumbai
19	PEG 400	S.D. Fine Chem. Ltd., Mumbai
20	Transcutol	Gattefosse Limited, France
21	Liquid filled capsules	ACG Capsules, Mumbai

22	Aerosil 200	Oxford Laboratory Reagent, Mumbai
23	Neusilin US2	Fuji Chemical Industry Co., Ltd., Japan
24	Crosscarmellose sodium	Alkem Laboratories, Navi Mumbai
25	Sodium starch glycolate	Alkem Laboratories, Navi Mumbai
26	Polyplasdone XL-10	Alkem Laboratories, Navi Mumbai
27	Microcrystalline cellulose	Anshul Agencies, Mumbai
28	Doshion P-544	Doshion Water Solution Pvt. Ltd., Ahmadabad
29	Methanol – AR Grade	Merck Chemicals, Mumbai
30	Ethanol– AR Grade	Merck Chemicals, Mumbai
31	Distilled water- HPLC grade	Merck Chemicals, Mumbai
32	Acetonitrile	Merck Chemicals, Mumbai - AR grade

Table 17. List of equipment / instrument used in present work

Sr. No.	Equipment/Instrument	Make & Model
1	Electronic Balance	Shimadzu, AUX200
2	UV Spectrophotometer	Jasco, Japan, V-630
3	FTIR Spectrophotometer	Jasco, Japan, M4100
4	Differential Scanning Calorimeter	Mettler Star SW9.20, DSC 6220
5	Ultrasonicator	Biomedica, BMI 599
5	Magnetic Stirrer	Remi, India, 1 MLH
6	Hot Air Oven	Biomedica, BM-D-45
7	Orbital shaker	Memmert, SV 1422, Germany
8	Melting point apparatus	Veego, India, VMP-I
9	Particle zeta sizer	Horiba SZ-100, Kyoto, Japan
10	pH meter	Equi-Tronics, EQ-610
11	Centrifuge machine	Remi, India
12	Compression machine	Rimek, Mini press-1
13	Bulk density test apparatus	Electrolab
14	Hardness Tester	Erweka TBH 125
15	Vernier Caliper	Mitutoyo-Digimatic
16	Disintegration test apparatus	Electrolab, EI 901
17	USP Dissolution test Apparatus	Electrolab, TDT-06L
18	Stability Chamber	Oswal's scientific, Fabricated

Software's used

Table 18. List of Software's used

Sr. No.	Name of software	Name of version
1	CHEMEX school	3.6
2	Design Expert	13
3	PCP Disso	V 2.08
4	Graph Prism	Version 7
5	PK solver	2.0

8. EXPERIMENTAL WORK

8.1. Preformulation studies of drug and excipients [119-121]

Pre-formulation studies are laboratorial investigations identifying active ingredients and excipient characteristics which can influence formulation, design and performance of the process. It was defined as "learning before doing." The physical-chemical characteristics of chemical or organic entities which may impact their evolution into finished products should be studied during various phases of development. Preformulation data are crucial for determining the potential and process limitations of human and animal pharmacokinetics while the product is increasing in production. Preformulation studies are also conducted in order to predict formulation stability throughout production, shipping and storage and therefore to determine the shelf life of the product supplied.

8.1.1. Organoleptic properties

The PZQ drug sample was manually analyzed for the organoleptic properties like color, odour, taste and appearance.

8.1.2. Melting point determination

Melting point of PZQ was determined by using melting point apparatus (Veego, VMP 1). Observed value was compared with the reported value.

8.1.3. Fourier Transform Infrared Spectra (FTIR) analysis

The IR spectra of PZQ was recorded by using Fourier Transform Infrared Spectrophotometer (Make: Jasco Japan M 4100) by using the Potassium bromide (KBr) pellet method and scanned in the range of 4000 to 400 cm^{-1}.

8.1.4. Differential Scanning Calorimetry (DSC)

Thermal analysis of PZQ was carried out by using Differential Scanning Calorimeter (Make: Mettler star, DSC 6220). Approximately 2 to 5 mg of sample was heated in a closed pierced aluminum pan from 20^0C to 200^0C at a heating rate of 10^0C/min under a stream of nitrogen.

8.1.5. Powder X-Ray Diffraction (PXRD) analysis

Powder X-ray diffraction (PXRD) spectra of PZQ was recorded by using an powder X-Ray diffractometer (Make: X-Ray generator Philips Ltd, Ru-200B) with Cu-Kα radiation (Voltage 40 kV and the current 30 mA). The scanning angle ranged from 5 to 25^0 of 2θ.

8.2. UV-Spectroscopy Study

8.2.1. Determination of λmax

A carefully weighed quantity (10 mg) of PZQ was dissolved in a methanol with a continuous stirring up to 100 ml to get stock solution of 100μg/ml. This solution was utilized as a reference and scanned with a UV/Visible spectrophotometer (Jasco, Japan, V-630) to methanol in the region between 200 and 400 nm. The λmax was determined.

8.2.2. Preparation of standard calibration curves

If the medication has an ultraviolet spectrum absorption range, UV spectroscopy may be utilized for quantitative examination. The law of Beer's states that absorption is proportional to the chemical concentration at a certain wavelength. The linear link between absorption and concentration advantages quantitative computations, for example solubility and drug release investigations. The beer curve offers an easy estimate of the chemical absorption concentration. A variety of media have calibrated the medication. The following are the information:

8.2.3. Calibration curve in different media (UV method)

Praziquentel, 10 mg has been properly weighed and mixed with adequate quantity of methanol, 0.1 N HCl, phosphate buffer pH-6.8 and phosphate buffer pH-7.4, in separate volume flasks to produce a volume of 100 ml. The consequence was a shaken dispersion. Further dilutions of 5-100 μg/ml were produced by using the appropriate solvents from this stock solution. The absorbance of these solutions was tested by using a UV-visible spectrophotometer at 263 nm.

8.3. Solubility studies

PZQ solubility in pure water and a variety of buffer solutions were studied (pH- 1.2, 6.8, 7.4). A 10 ml vial of each solvent was transferred to the screw-capped glass vial of 2 ml containing the excess medicine. The above mentioned solutions were first combined with the PZQ and the solvents were soniced. It kept for 72 hrs at 25±0.5°C mixes in a orbital shaker (Memmert, SV 1422, Germany). The mixture was then centrifuged for 30 minutes at 5000 rpm. A Millipore membrane filter (0.45 μm) was used to filter the supernatant solution, which was afterwards diluted with methanol at required quantities. UV-Visible (Jasco, Japan, V-630) spectrophotometer was used to detect PZQ in 263 nm using methanol as a blank. All measurements were done in triplicates. [122,123]

8.3.1. Solubility study of PZQ in various oils, surfactants and co-surfactants

In addition, the solubility of PZQ was assessed in several oils (Capmul MCM, Capryol 90, Oleic acid, Arachis oil, Captex 300, Castor oil, Soyabean oil, Isopropyl myristate, Labrafil, Olive oil & Almond oil), surfactants (Cremophore RH 40, Tweens 80, Tweens 20 & Span 20) and co-surfactants (PEG 400, Transcutol & Propylene glycol). The above mixtures were continuously mixed with the drug by using a magnetic stirrer (REMI 1 MLH) for around 2 minutes. These mixtures were stirred in an orbital shaker (Memmert, SV 1422, Germany) for 72 hours at 25±0.5°C and then kept 24 hours for equilibrium. The samples were then collected and centrifuged (REMI C-24 BL) 5000 rpm for 30 min. The supernatant solution, which was subsequently diluted with methanol at necessary concentrations, was filtered with a Millipore membrane filter (0.45 μm). A UV-Visible spectrophotometer (JASCO V-630) was used to measure the concentration of PZQ at 263 nm and a blank methanol was applied. Three times all measurements were acquired.

8.3.2. Preliminary screening of surfactants

For emulsification ability by utilizing the technique of Date and Nagarsenker, several surfactants were evaluated. The combination of surfactant and oil was 1:1. (300 mg of the surfactants, Cremophore RH 40, Tweens 80, Tweens 20 & Span 20 were added to 300 mg of the oily phase i.e. Capmul MCM). By heating the mixtures to 45-50°C, the components were homogenised. The fine-emulsion with double distilled water up to 50 ml has been diluting every 50 mg mixture in a stopped volumetric flask. The number of flask inversion needed to produce a homogenous emulsion has affected the ease of emulsification. It has been let to remain in a for 2 hours and % transmittance at 638.2 nm was evaluated by using UV Spectrophotometer (JASCO V-630). These emulsions were examined visually for any indication of phase separation or turbidity. [53]

8.3.3. Preliminary screening of co-surfactants

Several co-surfactants (PEG 400, Transcutol and Propylene glycol) have been evaluated by utilizing the chosen oily phase and surfactants at a ratio of 3.2:1. Combinations of 300 mg oil, 200 mg surfactant and 100 mg co-surfactant were produced and tested, similarly as above.

8.4. Construction of pseudo-ternary phase diagrams

On the basis of solubility studies and preliminary screening of surfactants and co-surfactants, Capmul MCM was selected as the oil, Cremophore RH 40 was selected as the surfactant and PEG400 was selected as co-surfactant. The oil quantity (X1) and the Smix ratio (X2) were the independent variables of the CCD. Oil, Smix and water were 100% concentrated in the three components. At desired (ratio of surfactant to co-surfactant) value (1:1, 2:1 and 3:1), oil and Smix were mixed at ratio of 1:9, 2:8, 3:7, 4:6, 5:5, 6:4, 7:3, 8:2 and 9:1. Based on early study findings, the X1 and X2 ranges were selected. In order to respond to all model formulations, the Design-Expert® tool was utilized (version 13). [124-126]

8.5. Experimental Design

A two-factor central composite design (CCD) was used for optimizing the composition of liquid SEDDS. In the CCD independent variable were oil (X1) and surfactant to co-surfactant ratio i.e. Smix (X2). The combined oil, surfactant and water concentration of the three components was 100%. Based on the early research results, the X1 and X2 ranges were chosen. The Design-Expert® programme (version 13) was used to address all model formulations. The independent variables and the corresponding CCD matrix technology are illustrated in Table 19 and 20 respectively.

Table 19. Experimental range and level of independent variables

Independent Variable	Unit	$-\alpha$	-1	0	+1	$+\alpha$
Oil (X_1)	%	5.85	10	20	30	34.14
S_{mix} Ratio (X_2)	-	0.585	1	2	3	3.414

Table 20. The 2 factor CCD matrix experimental values

Run	X1 Capmul MCM (%)	X2 (Cremophore RH-40:PEG400)
F1	20	61.85:18.14 (3.41:1)
F2	10	45:45 (1:1)
F3	20	53.4:26.6 (2:1)
F4	10	67.5:22.5 (3:1)
F5	20	29.36:50.63 (0.58:1)
F6	30	35:35 (1:1)
F7	5.85	62.76:31.38 (2:1)
F8	34.14	43.9:21.95 (2:1)
F9	30	52.5:17.5 (3:1)
F10	20	53.4:26.6 (2:1)
F11	20	53.4:26.6 (2:1)
F12	20	53.4:26.6 (2:1)
F13	20	53.4:26.6 (2:1)
F14	20	53.4:26.6 (2:1)

- **Independent variables**

  X1 = Oil (Capmul MCM C8) %

  X2= Smix (Cremophore RH-40:PEG400) Ratio

- **Dependent variables**

  Y1= % Transmittance

  Y2= Globule size

  Y3 = Self emulsification time

  Y4 = % Drug release

In order to evaluate the quality of SEDDS were used as responses (dependent variables) % transmittance (Y1), globule size (Y2), self-emulsification time (Y3) and % drug release (Y4). Multiple linear regression analysis evaluated the influence of factors on the response (MLRA). The best suitable mathematical model was selected by utilizing Design-Expert software to compare several statistical features such as standard deviation (SD), multiple correlation coefficients (R^2) and an adjusted coefficient of correlation (adjusted R^2). The CCD model has been constructed with the following multiple regression analysis equations to fit the second order polynomial model,

$$Y= b_0 + b_1 X_1+b_2X_2+ b3X^2_1+ b4X^2_2 + b_5 X_1X_2 \qquad \text{---------------} (2)$$

Where,

Y is the dependent variable (factor),

b_0 is the intercept,

X1and X2 correspond to the studied factors,

b_1-b_5 are the regression coefficients.

8.6. Formulation of liquid self-emulsifying formulation loaded with PZQ

The weighed amount of Smix, i.e. surfactant and co-surfactant, was combined in a vial on magnetic stirrer (Mixture-1). The estimated amount of PZQ was dissolved in a separate beaker in the calculated quantity of oil (Capmul MCM) (Mixture-2). The oil (Mixture-2) phase was put into the surfactant co-surfactant mixture (Mixture-1) drop by drop and mixed until liquid SEDDS was obtained.

8.7. Characterization of formulations [127-130]

8.7.1. Thermodynamic stability

a. Centrifugation stability

These formulations were centrifuged at 5000 rpm (REMI C-24 BL) for 30 minutes to assess system stability and were looking for cracking, drug precipitation, phase separation and creaming. For those compositions that were stable, the heating-cooling cycle was chosen.

b. Heating and cooling cycle

Three cycles between temperatures 4°C and 45°C, with storage duration not less than 48 hours per temperature. Those formulations, which were stable at these temperatures, were subjected to Freeze thaw test.

c. Freeze thaw cycle

The formulations had three freeze-thaw cycles between -20°C and +25 °C with a storage period not less than 48 hours at each temperature. These formulations were then evaluated visually for the separation of the phase. Those formulations that were stable for the phase separation were also adopted for the dispersibility test to evaluate the efficiency of self-emulsification.

8.7.2. Dispersibility test

For this, of each formulation (0.5 ml) was added drop by drop in each glass beaker with 250 ml of double distilled water, kept at 37^0 C ± 0.5^0 C at 100 rpm, by using hotplate magnetic stirrer (REMI 1 MLH). The time required for the SEDDS to vanish was noted. The effectiveness of SEDDS was visually assessed using the five grading method as shown in table 21.

Table 21. Grades of emulsions

Sr. No.	Dispersibility and appearance	Grade
1	Rapid forming microemulsion, (within 60 sec.) clear or slightly bluish in appearance	A
2	Rapidly forming (within 2 min.), slightly less clear emulsion, having a bluish white appearance	B
3	Fine emulsion but milky appearance (within 120 sec.)	C
4	Dull, grayish white emulsion with a slightly oily appearance (longer than 120 sec.)	D
5	Exhibit either poor or minimal emulsification with large oil globules (longer than 180 sec.)	E

8.7.3. Robustness to dilution

Robustness to dilution was studied by diluting the formulation 50, 100 and 1000 times with different diluents i.e. double distilled water, 0.1 N HCl and phosphate buffer pH 6.8. The diluted samples were stored for 24 h and observed for any signs of physical changes.

8.7.4. Transmission electron microscopy

Transmission electron microscopy was performed for visual inspection by an optimized batch of liquid SEDDS (F7). The picture was captured with an transmission electron microscope.

8.7.5. Transmittance test

The stability of SEDDS formulation on dilution was tested using a UV-visible spectrophotometer (JASCO, V-630) to determine the transmittance where distilled water served as blank. The each sample transmittance was measured at 638.2 nm.

8.7.6. Determination of self-emulsification time

For each formulation (1 ml) was added to 900 ml of distilled water under continuous stirring (50 rpm), by using USP type-II dissolution apparatus at 37±0.5°C. The time required for distributing in the system entirely and the time for emulsification was recorded in seconds

8.7.7. Cloud point measurement

Every formulation was diluted by distilling water to a ratio of 1:250 and placed in a water bath at a continuously rising temperature. The point at which cloudiness occurs was designated as a cloud point.

8.7.8. Globule size determination

By using the photon correlation spectroscopy (Horiba SZ-100, Kyoto, Japan) mean globule size and polydispersity index of the resultant emulsions were measured. The sample temperature was fixed at 25°C and detection was carried out a scattering angle of 90°.

8.7.9. Determination of zeta potential

The Zeta potential was determined by using photon correlation spectroscopy.

8.7.10. Determination of drug content

The P-L-SEDDS formulations (1 ml) have been dissolved in 10 ml of methanol by using sonicator for 5 min. Subsequently, then solution was filtered, diluted appropriately and the PZQ content was analyzed spectrophotometrically.

8.7.11. *In-vitro* dissolution studies

In-vitro drug release test was performed by using a USP Type-II dissolution test apparatus (Electrolab and TDT), in a 900 ml 0.1N HCl at 37±0.5°C. 5 ml aliquots were taken at intervals of 0, 2, 5, 10, 15, 20, 25, 30, 45 and 60 min. and replaced with a new dissolving media in the same amount. After filtration through 0.45 μm pore sized membrane filter, appropriately diluted with methanol and analysis was carried out by using UV method.

8.7.12. Stability study

The stability test was assessed according to the requirements of ICH Q 1 A (R2) the stability assessment of new pharmaceutical substances and products. The capsules were filled with liquid-SEDDS (F7), wrapped with aluminium strips and kept in air-tight glass containers and protected from light. At 0, 1, 2, 3 and 6 months, temperature and humidity control were maintained under accelerated circumstances ($40^0C \pm 2^0C$, 75±5% RH). The appearance, self-emulsifying characteristics, drug content and centrifugation test of liquid-SEDDS were evaluated. [131,132]

8.8. Anthelmintic Activity [133, 134]

8.8.1. Collection of earthworms

Earthworms were spotted in a marshy region near Otur, Pune, India. Earthworms size ranged between 5 to 8 cm. Due to its anatomical and physiological resemblance to intestinal round worms and parasites of human beings were used *in-vitro* to evaluate anthelmintic activity.

8.8.2. Evaluation of anthelmintic activity by using earthworms

In a petridish with 10 ml of optimized liquid SEDDS (F7), earthworms were kept with an average length 5 to 8 cm, at temperatures of 37°C. This was done by emptying petri plates into a wash basin and allowing the worms to move freely. These worms were paralyzed and exhibited a lack of motion in the solution. There were measurements of how long it took to paralyze the worms and perish.

8.9. Formulation of solid SEDDS [135, 136]

The optimized liquid SEDDS formulation (F7) was converted into free flowing powders by using adsorbents, such as aerosil 200 and Neusilin US2. The optimized liquid SEDDS was added dropwise into the solid adsorbent and mixed with a mortar and pestle.

8.9.1. Precompression evaluation parameters of powder blend [136, 137]

1) Bulk Density (BD)

Bulk density is defined as the mass of a powder to the bulk volume. The following formula was used to determine the bulk density (ρb):

$$\text{Bulk density } (\rho b) = \frac{\text{Weight of powder (M)}}{\text{Bulk volume (Vb)}} \qquad \text{-------------- (3)}$$

2) Tapped Density (TD)

It is the ratio of the total powder mass to the tapped powder volume. By applying the following formula the tapped density (ρt) was obtained:

$$\text{Tapped density } (\rho t) = \frac{\text{Weight of powder (M)}}{\text{Tapped volume (Vt)}} \qquad \text{-------------- (4)}$$

3) Carr's Index

The % Carr's Index (I) of the powder was determined by using the following formula,

% Carr's index (I) = {(Tapped density – Bulk density) / Tapped density} X 100 ------ (5)

4) Hausner's ratio

Hausner's ratio is an indirect index of ease of powder flow. It was calculated by the following formula,

$$\text{Hausner's ratio} = \frac{\text{Tapped density } (\rho t)}{\text{Bulk density } (\rho b)} \qquad \text{-------- (6)}$$

5) Angle of repose

The angle of repose was calculated by using the following formula,

$$\text{Angle of repose } (\theta) = \tan^{-1} \frac{\text{height (h)}}{\text{radius (r)}} \qquad \text{--------- (7)}$$

8.10. Solid state characterization of S-SEDDS

8.10.1. Fourier Transform Infrared Spectra (FTIR) analysis

The IR-spectrum for optimized S-SEDDS was recorded with a Potassium Bromide (KBr) pellet technique by utilizing the Fourier Transform Infrared Spectrophotometer (Make: Jasco, Japan, M 4100) and was scanned between 4000 and 400 cm^{-1}. The spectra obtained for PZQ and P-S-SEDDS were compared.

8.10.2. Differential Scanning Colorimetry (DSC)

Thermal analysis of optimized S-SEDDS was conducted with differential scanning calorimeter (DSC). In the set temperature of 20°C to 200°C, a heating rate of 10°C/min was used, in an inert nitrogen environment.

8.10.3. Powder X-Ray Diffraction (PXRD) analysis

Powder X-ray diffraction (PXRD) study was studied by using an X-ray diffractometer with Cu-Kα radiation (Voltage 40 kV and the current 30 mA). The scanning angle ranged from 5 to 25^0 of 2θ.

8.10.4. Scanning electron microscope analysis

A small amount of powder was mounted on stab. SEM micrograph of the surfaces of the S-SEDDS powder was photographed by using scanning electron microscope.

8.11. Formulation and development of solid self-emulsifying drug delivery system (S-SEDDS) tablets

The S-SEDDS tablets were prepared by using a direct compression method using several superdisintegrants including sodium starch glycolate, Crosscarmellose sodium and polyplasdone XL-10 at different dose as described in Table 22. S-SEDDS, povidone, microcrystalline cellulose, mannitol, magnesium stearate, doshion P-544 and aspartame, all accurately weighed prior to the combination and all the materials were screened by a 60 # screen. The final powder was compressed into tablets by using a rotary tablet machine. The 3^2 factorial design was applied for the S-SEDDS tablet formulation of Praziquantel. [138]

Table 22. Formulation of 3^2 factorial design for Praziquantel S-SEDDS

Ingredients (mg)	T1	T2	T3	T4	T5	T6	T7	T8	T9
S-SEDDS	160	160	160	160	160	160	160	160	160
Sodium starch Glycolate	7.5	10	12.5	--	--	--	--	--	--
Crosscarmellose sodium	--	--	--	7.5	10	12.5	--	--	--
Polyplasdone XL-10	--	--	--	--	--	--	7.5	10	12.5
Povidone	7.5	7.5	7.5	7.5	7.5	7.5	7.5	7.5	7.5
Microcrystalline cellulose	25	25	25	25	25	25	25	25	25
Mannitol	34	31.5	29	34	31.5	29	34	31.5	29
Magnesium Stearate	2.5	2.5	2.5	2.5	2.5	2.5	2.5	2.5	2.5
Doshion P-544	12.5	12.5	12.5	12.5	12.5	12.5	12.5	12.5	12.5
Aspartame	1	1	1	1	1	1	1	1	1
Total (mg)	**250**	**250**	**250**	**250**	**250**	**250**	**250**	**250**	**250**

8.12. Evaluation of tablets [139, 140]

8.12.1. Hardness

The hardness of the tablet of each formulation was determined by using the Monsanto Hardness tester.

8.12.2. Thickness

The thickness was measured by using Digital Vernier calipers.

8.12.3. Friability

This test will assess capacity of tablets can withstand abrasion during packing, handling and transport. To determine friability by using the Roche friabilator, the following formula is employed,

$$\% \text{ Friability} = \frac{\text{Loss in weight}}{\text{Initial weight}} \times 100 \quad \text{------- (8)}$$

Where, Loss in weight = weight of tablets before test - weight of tablets after test

8.12.4. Uniformity of weight

The average weight of the tablet was calculated from collective weight according to Indian Pharmacopoeia method.

8.12.5. Drug content

The accurate weight of powder was dissolved in 0.1 N HCl with 2 mg per ml of sodium lauryl sulphate, the solution was properly filtered and diluted. UV-visible spectrometer was used for analyzing drug content at 263 nm.

8.12.6. *In-vitro* drug release study

The USP type-II device was used for the research of *in-vitro* drug releases. The dissolution test was performed by using 900 ml 0.1 N HCl with per ml of 2 mg sodium lauryl sulphate as the dissolution media at 37°C±0.5°C. 5 ml aliquots, at intervals of 2, 5, 10, 15, 20, 25 and 30 minutes, were withdrawn, filtered and replaced with 5 ml of fresh dissolution medium. The % drug release was measured by using a UV-Visible spectrometer at 263 nm.

8.12.7. Comparison of *In-vitro* dissolution study of a prepared tablet with marketed formulation

In-vitro dissolution research is used to compare a produced tablet with the marketed tablet formulation. (Distoside Tablet).

8.12.8. Similarity factor

The *in vitro* dissolution data of the optimized tablet formulation and marketed tablet formulation studies was compared by using similarity factor f_2. The optimized tablet formulation was considered as test formulation and Marketed formulation was considered as reference formulation. Dissolution profiles are considered as similar if f_2 value is found in between 50-100.

8.12.9. Stability Study

The stability study was carried out an optimized tablet formulation according to ICH guidelines. An accelerated stability study was carried out at 40°C±2°C, 75% ±5% RH with temperature and humidity control were measurements at 1, 2, 3 and 6 months was undertaken. The tablets of the optimized formulation were packaged into HDPE (High Density Polyethylene) containers and stored in a stability chamber. The samples were evaluated at regular intervals for physical appearance, disintegration time, globule size, zeta potential, drug content and drug release.

8.13. Taste masking approach

The complexity of resins with ion exchanges has shown that they mask the bitter taste of a broad variety of drugs as a simple and cost effective process. This method essentially binding bitter matter to a resin substrate which is counter loaded and thus creates a complex for the drug-resin. The material nearly completely decomposes due to the heavy concentration of hydrogen ions in the gastrointestinal tract. Into the intestine, hydrogen ions or ion exchange ions disintegrate the resin medication structure, causing the complex and subsequent release into the gastric contents to be increased elution or decay. The free medicine is now available and can be safely swallowed via the gastrointestinal tract. The flavour of a medicine may also be masked without damaging its absorption. The compound is disguised by the complexation of Doshion P-544 DS resin by means of an ion exchange complexation.

Bitter taste is quantified by the impressions of volunteers about the bitter human taste. The preparation process was outlined to the volunteers and a permission statement was requested to be signed. Per volunteer maintained 15 seconds in their mouth a 20 mg suspension of Praziquantel compared with the formulation.

8.14. Bioanalytical Method development

A Bioanalytical approach was created for the optimized Praziquantel S-SEDDS tablet to assess several pharmacokinetic parameters after ingestment of the optimized Praziquantel tablet (T3).

8.14.1. Experimental animals

In vivo study was conducted in accordance with the Committee for the Purpose of Control and Supervision of Experiments on Animals (CPCSEA, Government of India) guidelines and approved by Institutional Animal Ethics Committee (IAEC), - Gourishankar Institute of Pharmaceutical Education and Research, Limb, Satara (Approval No. GIPER/IAEC/2020-21/02). In this experiment, healthy white albino rats (weighing 150±20 grams) were used. The rats were bought from prestigious local retailers and are maintained in the Pharmaceutical Education and Research Institute of Gourishankar in Limb, Satara-415004. The cage was maintained at 25°C constantly. The venous blood samples (0.2 mL) were collected in a heparinized-coated micro-centrifuge tube with the retro orbital plexus of albino rats with a capacity of 2 mL. Different intervals of the samples were taken: 0, 0.15, 0.5, 1, 2, 4, 8, 12, 20, 24 hours following dosing. These samples were then centrifuged at 12000 rpm for 15 minutes and the plasma was extracted very carefully. Each heparinized tube containing sample preparation was administered 8.25% perchloric acid to precipitate plasma protein. The graph between time and the measured plasma concentration was produced after calculation of the pharmacokinetic parameters. The area under curve (AUC) was calculated by using the linear trapezoidal technique. Some pharmacokinetic parameters have been observed, such as concentration (Cmax), the time at which Cmax was observed (Tmax) etc. [141,142]

8.14.1.1. Animals required for study

Table 23. Animals required for study

a. Species / Common name	**White albino rats**
b. Age / Weight / Size	150 ± 20 gm
c. Gender	Male
d. No. to be used	12
e. Purpose of animal use	*In-vivo* study of solid self emulsifying drug delivery system

8.14.1.2. Reagents and chemicals

Praziquantel, Diazepam, Acetonitrile, Methanol, Perchloric acid, water.

Table 24. List of Chemicals

Name of the Chemical	CAS Number	Grade
Praziquantel	55268-74-1	AR Grade
Diazepam	439-14-5	AR Grade
Acetonitrile	75-05-8	HPLC Grade
Methanol	67-56-1	HPLC Grade
Perchloric acid	7601-90-3	AR Grade

8.14.1.3. Instruments

Jasco PU-2085 Plus with quaternary gradient pump was used for method development by using UV/VIS detector. By using chromatopro software, the HPLC system was built. Analysis of HPLC was done using a column of Hypersil ODS C18 (average particle size 5 mm) column (250 mm, 4.6 mm).\

8.14.1.4. Mobile Phase

The mobile phase consisted of Acetonitrile-Methanol-Water (50:10:40 v/v). The eluent was monitored with the UV detector at 217 nm with a flow rate of 1 mL/min and sample size of 20 μl was carried out. For filtration 0.45 μm membrane filter was used.

Table 25. HPLC System Parameters

Column	C18
Mobile Phase Ratio	50:10:40 v/v
Mobile Phase	Acetonitrile-Methanol-Water
Flow Rate	1 ml/min
Wavelength	217 nm
Drug	Praziquantel
Sample Size	20 μl
Retention Time	6.41 min

8.14.1.5. Selection of Mobile Phase

For selecting mobile extraction by using various solvents have been selected in order to discover the appropriate mobile phase for the bioanalytical technique. Extraction was performed with Methanol, Acetonitrile and Water.

8.14.1.6. Preparation of rat plasma sample preparation

1. Praziquantel was isolated from plasma in the rat by using the liquid-liquid extraction method.

2. Upon oral administration of Praziquantel S-SEDDS tablet at 20 mg/kg dosing then blood samples were collected. Before administering the animals were kept fasted for overnight (~12 hr.). During fasting animals had free access to water.

3. Blood samples (0.2 mL) were collected and placed in heparin covered perchloric acid tube for plasma protein precipitation. Samples of retro orbital plexus 0, 0.15, 0.5, 1, 2, 4, 8, 12, 20 and 24 hours were taken and vortexed at 12000 rpm for 15 minutes by centrifugation. After samples were collected.

4. Simultaneously in 1.5 ml of centrifugal tubes with diazepam and a blank (200 µl of plasma without Praziquantel and Diazepam), at a fixed concentration.

5. These samples then transferred into auto sampler vials for injection.

8.14.1.7. Preparation of standard stock solutions

1. A stock solution of 1mg/ml praziquantel and diazepam were prepared in methanol.

2. Mix and dilute the standard solution of praziquantel and diazepam in the same amount of a individual stock solution of methanol.

3. The final concentration varied from 10, 50, 100, 500, 1000, 1300 and 1500 ng/ml for the standard solution.

4. A concentration set at 500 ng/ml of diazepam (internal standard) was used.

5. Different concentrations of 100, 500 and 1000 ng/ml with the constant IS concentration (500 ng/ml) were generated by using the same procedure.

6. Prior to each analysis and validation, a new fresh standard solution was prepared.

8.14.1.8. Preparation of Sample solution

1. 20 S-SEDDS tablets were accurately weighed and triturated in a mortar and pestle.

2. Praziquantel powder was weighed properly and put in a 100 ml flask.

3. Mobile phase of 80 mL were added, which were sonicated for a period of 15 minutes.

4. Using this mobile phase, the final volume was made up to 100 mL and the solution was filtered with a membrane filter of 0.22 µm.

5. This filtrate was further diluted to yield concentration of 100 µg/ml Praziquantel.

6. A linear trapezoidal rule was used to determine the total area under curve (AUC) verses time.

7. For the calculation of r^2 and the linear regression equation, this data was used.

8.14.1.9. Linearity

To verify the linearity of the method, a standard solution was prepared by using Praziquantel 100 ng/ml-1500 ng/ml. After injection, peak regions were used to construct the calibration curves against the concentrations.

8.14.2. Method validation

The International Conference on Harmonization and the United States Pharmacopeia issued guidelines for method validation. The following parameters were used to validate the suggested method. As per the ICH guidelines of the proposed bioanalytical HPLC technique validated for linearity, system suitability, specificity, precision and robustness.

8.14.2.1. Linearity

The ratio of peak areas of Praziquantel to Diazepam (Internal Standard) at various concentrations of Praziquantel. The chromatographic responses (ratio of peak areas of Praziquantel to Diazepam IS versus Praziquantel concentration) were checked for linearity over an analytical range of 100.0–1500.0 ng/ml.

8.14.2.2. System Suitability

Praziquantel with 100 ng/ml concentrations in six replicates, standard solutions were injected into the HPLC system. The standard solutions have been identified by using chromatographic parameters such as Rt values and peak areas. Then results showed that the suitability of the system for analysis.

8.14.2.3. Specificity

Praziquantel solutions with 100 µg/ml concentrations have been injected duplicates in the case of blank, standard and sample solutions. The specificity of the technique was assessed by comparing chromatograms obtained for all solutions.

8.14.2.4. Method precision

Praziquantel sample solutions with a dose of 100 µg/ml were injected in 6 replicates and analyzed for drug content. The % assay was calculated and the findings reported as a % relative standard deviation for both analysts.

8.14.2.5. Robustness

In order to demonstrate the robustness of the bioanalytical technology, the effects of changes in chromatographic conditions were evaluated according to ICH principles. Changes have been taken into account in the flow rate and content of mobile phases. The retention time for praziquantel and % RSD for each chromatographic condition was calculated.

9. RESULTS AND DISCUSSION

9.1. Preformulation study

9.1.1. Organoleptic properties

Organoleptic properties are given below table 26.

Table 26. Organoleptic properties of PZQ

Organoleptic properties	Inference
Colour	White
Odor	Odourless
Taste	Slightly bitter
Appearance	Crystalline powder

9.1.2. Melting point determination

The melting point is known as the temperature at which a material balances its solid and liquid phases. The reported and observed melting values were virtually the same and confirmed the purity of sample. A pure material has a sharp melting point where as impure material shows broad range melting point. The melting point is therefore utilized as a characterization method in preformulation research. Praziquantel melting point was detected at 140°C and a reported value of 136-141°C.

9.1.3. FTIR

Identification of pure drug was carried out by using Fourier Transform Infra-red Spectrophotometry (Jasco, Japan, M4100). The pure drug Praziquantel exhibited sharp peak at 3287.07 cm−1, 3003.59 cm−1, 2925.48 cm−1, 1630 cm−1, 1443.46 cm−1, 1350 cm−1 and 1126.22 cm−1 indicating the presence of O-H stretching, C-H stretching aromatic, C-H stretching alkyl, C=O stretching, C-C aromatic, C-N stretching and C-H bending, which confirms and identifies the drug when compared with the standard spectra of Praziquantel as shown in figure 1.

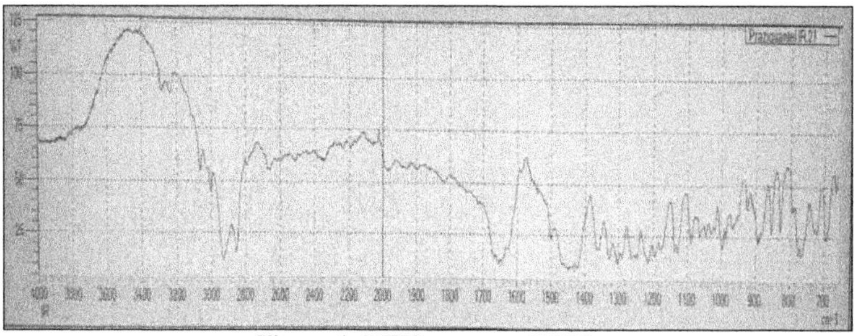

Figure 1. FTIR spectra of PZQ

9.1.4. DSC study

DSC is the useful method for the quantitative detection of all processes in which energy is required or produced. The DSC thermogram of PZQ as shown in Figure 2. Pure drug substance shows a sharp endothermic peak at 140^{0}C corresponding to its melting point.

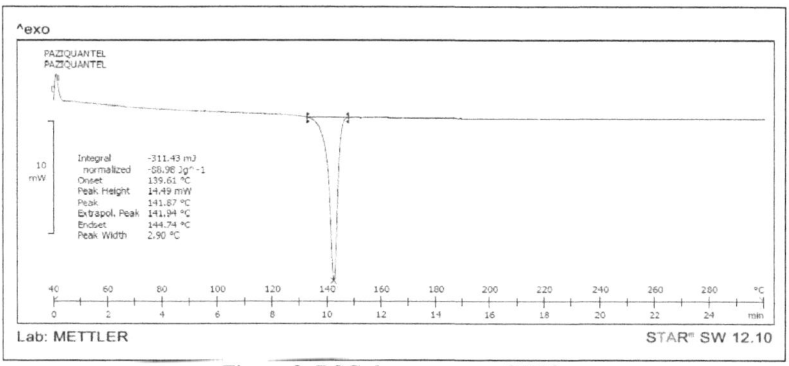

Figure 2. DSC thermogram of PZQ

9.1.5. Powder X-ray diffraction (PXRD) analysis

In case of crystalline material the X-rays undergo constructive and destructive interferences. The diffraction depends on particle shape and size of the material. PXRD studies of Praziquantel pure drug showed several sharp peaks at 5-25$^0\theta$ indicating crystalline nature as shown in figure 3.

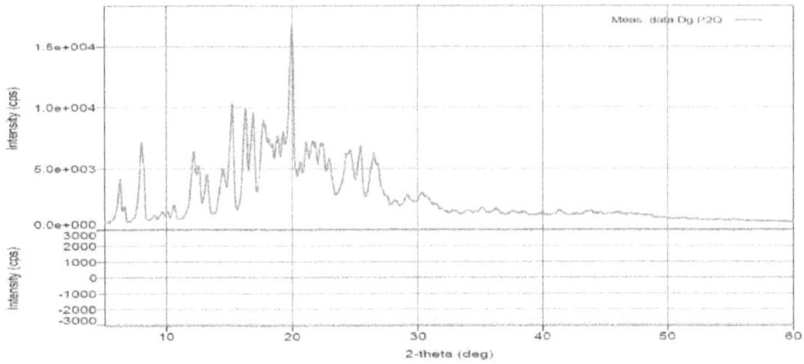

Figure 3. XRD spectra of PZQ

9.2. Preparation of calibration curve

Praziquentel showed highest absorption at 263 nm (λmax) as shown in graph 1. Hence 263 nm was selected as wavelength for obtaining calibration curve for Praziquentel.

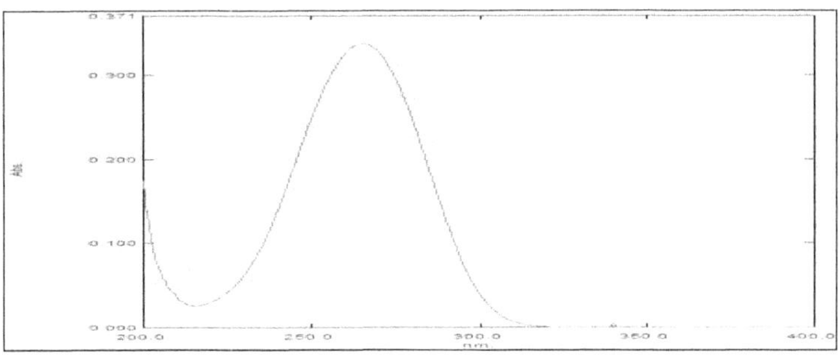

Graph 1. Determination of λmax of PZQ in methanol

9.2.1. Calibration curve in Methanol (UV method)

The results are summarized in the table 27. The regression coefficient for the calibration curve was found to be 0.999 and linearity was found in the range of 5 μg/ml to100 μg/ml.

Table 27. Absorbance data in Methanol

Concentration (µg/ml)	Absorbance (263 nm)
0	0
10	0.075
20	0.132
40	0.255
60	0.374
80	0.491
100	0.608

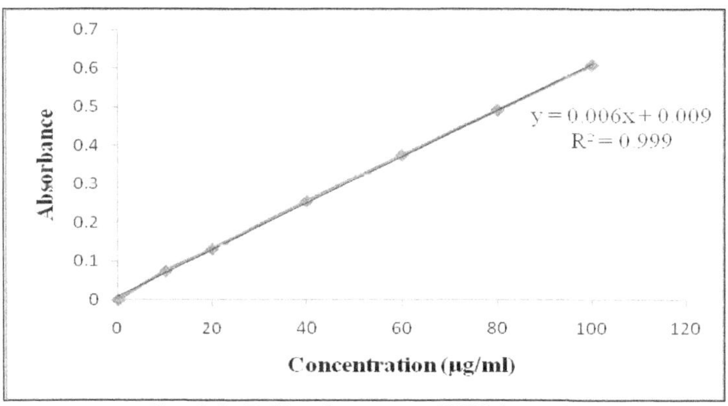

Graph 2. Calibration curve of PZQ in methanol

9.2.2. Calibration curve in 6.8 pH phosphate buffer

Table 28. Absorbance data in 6.8 pH phosphate buffer

Concentration (μg/ml)	Absorbance (263 nm)
0	0
5	0.038
10	0.071
20	0.135
40	0.313
60	0.475
80	0.643

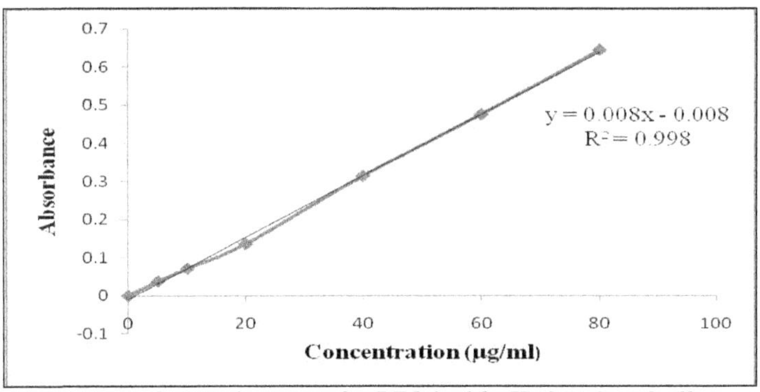

Graph 3. Calibration curve for PZQ in 6.8 pH phosphate buffer

The regression coefficient for the calibration curve was found to be 0.998 and linearity was found in the range of 5 μg/ml to 80 μg/ml.

9.2.3. Calibration curve in 7.4 pH phosphate buffer

Table 29. Absorbance data in 7.4 pH phosphate buffer

Concentration (µg/ml)	Absorbance(263 nm)
0	0
5	0.031
10	0.075
20	0.141
40	0.316
60	0.477
80	0.647

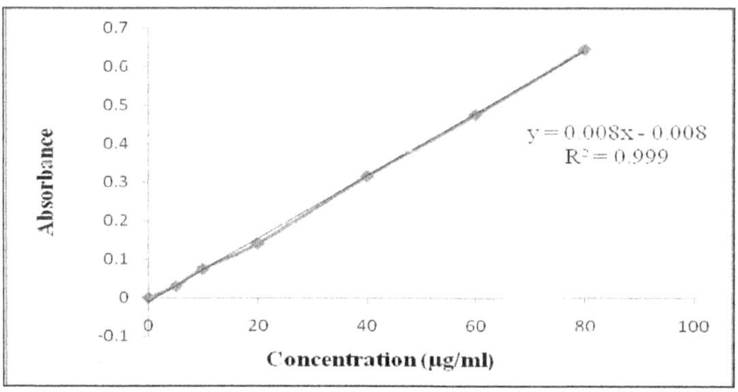

Graph 4. Calibration curve for PZQ in 7.4 pH Phosphate buffer

The regression coefficient for the calibration curve was found to be 0.999 and linearity was found in the range of 5 µg/ml to 80 µg/ml.

9.2.4. Calibration curve in 0.1 N HCl

Table 30. Absorbance data in 0.1 N HCl

Concentration (µg/ml)	Absorbance(263 nm)
0	0
5	0.029
10	0.065
20	0.149
40	0.32
60	0.481
80	0.648

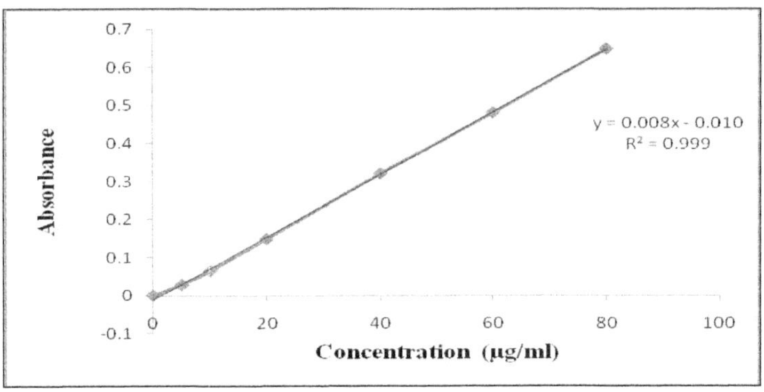

Graph 5. Calibration curve for chlorthalidone in 0.1 N HCl

The regression coefficient for the calibration curve was found to be 0.999 and linearity was found in the range of 5 µg/ml to 80 µg/ml.

9.3. pH dependent solubility

The solubility of PZQ in various solvents is indicated in table 31.

Table 31. Aqueous & pH dependent solubility data of PZQ (n=3)

Sr. No.	Solvents	Solubility(mg/ml)
1	Distilled Water	0.27 ± 0.07
2	pH 1.2	0.40 ± 0.05
3	pH 6.8	0.30 ± 0.08
4	pH 7.4	0.29 ± 0.07

9.4. Development of self-emulsifying drug delivery system (SEDDS)

SEDDS increases *in vitro* performance of the poor water soluble drugs and is therefore it serves as a suitable carrier to the administration of biopharmaceutical classification systems (BCS) belonging to Classes II and IV. The current study was performed to define the role of self-emulsifying formulations to enhance the solubility and bioavailability of the anthelmintic drug Praziquantel.

9.5. Solubility study

As many formulations undergo precipitation before undergoing in-situ solubilization, excipient solubility of a medication plays an essential role in influencing the stability of the formulations. Furthermore, while formulating PZQ loaded with SEDDS the entire PZQ dose should be soluble in SEDDS. Table 32 & 33 shows the solubility of PZQ in different oils, surfactants and co-surfactants. Among various vehicles screened, Capmul MCM was selected as the oil phase showing the highest solubilization capacity (57.94±0.70 mg/ml). Similarly, Cremophore RH40 (95.09±0.75 mg/ml) was used as surfactant & PEG 400 (70.49±0.84 mg/ml) was chosen as co-surfactant.

Table 32. Solubility of PZQ in various oils

Sr. No.	Oils	Solubility (mg/ml)
1	Capmul MCM	57.94 ± 0.70
2	Capryol 90	46.18 ± 1.80
3	Oleic acid	29.34 ± 0.67
4	Arachis oil	18.67 ± 0.49
5	Captex 300	11.20 ± 1.09
6	Castor oil	8.87 ± 0.33
7	Soyabean oil	5.44 ± 1.04
8	Isopropyl Myristate	4.29 ± 0.57
9	Labrafil	3.62 ± 0.43
10	Olive oil	3.41 ± 0.48
11	Almond oil	2.14 ± 0.55

Data expressed as mean ± SD (n = 3)

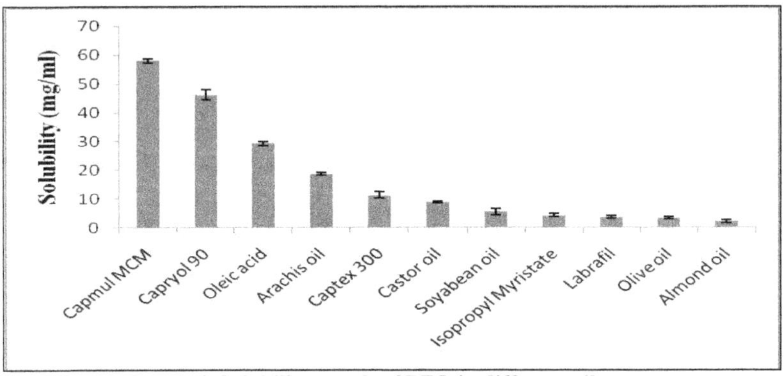

Graph 6. Solubility graph of PZQ in different oils

Table 33. Solubility of PZQ in various surfactants & co-surfactants

Sr. No.	Surfactants & Co-surfactants	Solubility (mg/ml)
1	Cremophore RH40	95.09 ± 0.75
2	Tween 80	38.78 ±0.71
3	Tween 20	8.92 ± 0.32
4	Span 20	6.65 ± 0.27
5	PEG 400	70.49 ± 0.84
6	Transcutol	20.66 ±0.95
7	Propylene glycol	12.11 ± 1.00

Data expressed as mean ± SD (n = 3)

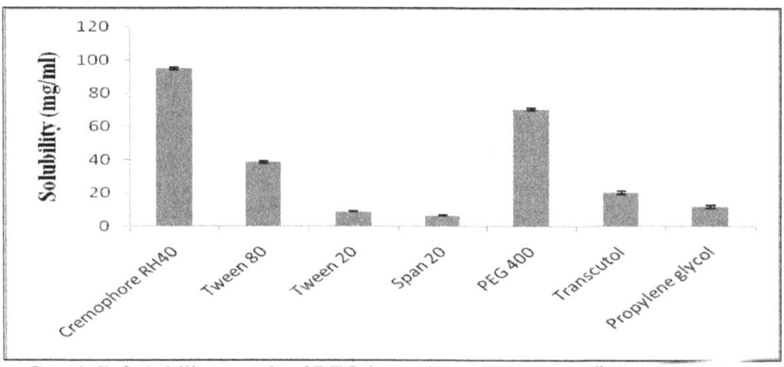

Graph 7. Solubility graph of PZQ in various surfactants & co-surfactants

9.5.1. Preliminary screening of surfactants for their emulsification ability

Under mild agitation condition, well-formulated SEDDS were disperse in seconds. The data indicate in table 34 that the highest transmittance, i.e. highest emulsification efficiency, is acquired by the following order Cremophore RH 40 > Tween 80 > Tween 20 > Span 20. The Cremophore RH 40 possessed the highest transmittance value and Span 20 as the lowest value.

Table 34. Emulsification ability of selected surfactants by using Capmul MCM as an oily phase

Sr. No.	Surfactants	Number of inversion	%Transmittance
1	Cremophore RH40	3.00 ±1.00	99.73 ± 0.44
2	Tween 80	5.33±0.577	89.3 ± 0.86
3	Tween 20	7.33±0.57	82.76 ± 1.20
4	Span 20	19.33±1.52	51.38 ± 1.51

Data expressed as mean ± SD (n = 3)

9.5.2. Preliminary screening of co-surfactants

This research compares three co-surfactants PEG 400, transcutol and propylene glycol. As shown in table 35, the transmittance of Capmul MCM as an oil and Cremophor RH40 as surfactant with all cosurfactants in the following sequence was outstanding: 99.60% PEG 400 > 97.16% of transcutol > 92.87% of propylene glycol. PEG 400 have been selected as the co-surfactant based on preliminary test results.

Table 35. Emulsification ability of selected Co-surfactants by using Capmul MCM as an oily phase and Cremophore RH40 as a Surfactant phase

Sr. No.	Co-surfactants	Number of inversion	%Transmittance
1	PEG 400	3.33±1.52	99.60 ± 0.28
2	Transcutol	11.66±1.04	97.16 ± 1.52
3	Propylene glycol	15±1.00	92.87 ± 1.73

Data expressed as mean ± SD (n = 3)

9.6. Construction of pseudo-ternary phase diagrams

Oil, water and Smix are the three corners of the fundamental schematic of the pseudoternary phase diagrams and total upto 100%. The combination of surfactant-cosurfactant mixture is known as Smix. Campul MCM as oil, Cremophore RH40 as surfactant and PEG 400 as co-surfactant were used for creating different phase diagrams, based on the findings of solubility study and preliminary examination of surfactants and cosurfactants.

The pseudo-ternary phase diagram consisting of (Capmul MCM + Cremophore RH40 + PEG 400) is as shown in figure 4 (A), (B) and (C) in a range of surfactant-co-surfactant ratios of 1:1, 2:1, and 3:1. respectively. The shaded region refers to a micro/nanoemulsion zone, whereas the wider area refers to more potential for self-emulsifying ability.

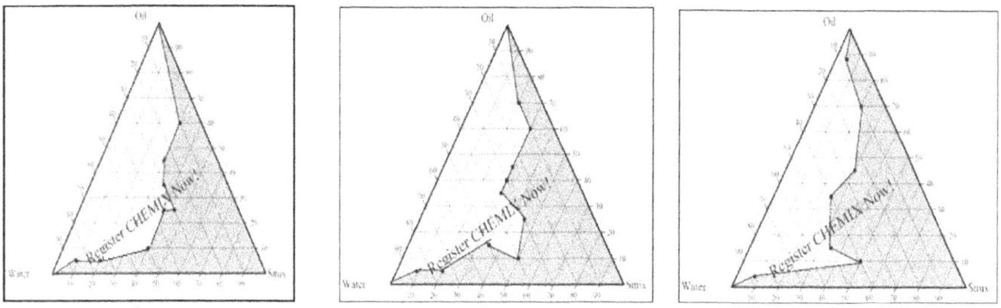

A B C

Figure 4. Pseudo ternary phase diagram with Capmul MCM (oil) & Cremophore RH40/PEG400 (Smix) in different ratio A) 1:1 B) 2:1 C) 3:1

9.7. Preliminary Batches evaluation

Preliminary batches were prepared as per table and their results are given in table 36.

Table 36: Evaluation of Thermodynamic stability and dispersion study of preliminary batches

Formulation code	Centrifugation	Heating and cooling	Freeze thaw	Dispersion	
				Grade	Inference
1	Passed	Passed	Passed	A	Passed
2	Passed	Passed	Passed	A	Passed
3	Passed	Passed	Passed	B	Passed
4	Passed	Passed	Passed	A	Passed
5	Passed	Passed	Passed	A	Passed
6	Passed	Passed	Passed	A	Passed
7	Passed	Passed	Passed	A	Passed
8	Passed	Passed	Passed	B	Passed
9	Passed	Passed	Passed	D	Fail
10	Passed	Passed	Passed	E	Fail

11	Fail	Fail	Fail	-	-
12	Fail	Fail	Fail	-	-
13	Fail	Fail	Fail	-	-
14	Fail	Fail	Fail	-	-

9.7.1. Thermodynamic stability studies

SEDDS are stable thermodynamic frames which pass this test exhibit no phase separation, creaming or cracking. Therefore, formulations were subjected to various thermodynamic tests, including centrifugation, heating and cooling cycles and freeze-thaw cycles to evaluate their stability. For dispersibility study, only stable formulations were used.

9.7.2. Dispersibility study

SEDDS should disperse completely and quickly when exposed to dilution under gentle agitation produced by peristaltic GIT activity. The easy water penetration of the colloidal phases produced on the droplet surface was thought to be related with the emulsification rate. A dispersibility test was conducted by using double distilled water. The formulations with grades A or B have been evaluated for future research. Those formulations failing Grade C, D and E dispersibility tests have been rejected for further research.

9.7.3. Robustness to dilution

SEDDS should create a homogeneous emulsion. Many dilution factors were used in various mediums for the formulations. All formulations which passed the dispersibility test and the reconstituted emulsion were not shown to have a precipitation, cloudiness or separation indications. This revealed that the SEDDS were robust to dilutions by fluids of different pH.

9.8. Optimization of P-L-SEDDS

In order to get the optimal P-L-SEDDS, CCD was applied in this study. For SEDDS system, it was expected that the

1) Maximum % transmittance produces clear and transparent solution.
2) Globule size should be minimum, so as to have better permeation.
3) Short self emulsification time for spontaneous emulsification.
4) Prompt drug release to give immediate effect.

Capmul MCM and Smix (Cremophore RH40:PEG400) were chosen as CCD independent variables, whereas dependent variables were % transmittance (Y1), globule size (Y2), self emulsification time (Y3) and % drug release (Y4). Table 37 presents the results of a total of eight different experimental runs. The impact of independent variables on the responses is depicted as 3D-Response surface plots and counter plots as shown in figure 5 and figure 6 respectively, while estimated regression coefficients (R^2), adjusted R^2 and regression (P-value and F-value) are given in table 38.

Table 37. Characterization Parameters of P-L-SEDDS Formulations

Formulations	% Transmittance± S.D.	Self emulsification time (Sec.) ± S.D.	Globule size (nm) ± S.D.	PDI ± S.D.	Zeta potential (mv) ± S.D.	Drug Content (%) ± S.D.	Cloud Point (°C) ± S.D.
F1	98.67 ± 0.64	50.66 ± 1.15	28.1 ± 0.75	0.330 ± 0.0062	-26.46 ± 1.28	98.96 ± 0.20	83.8 ± 1.00
F2	99.16 ± 0.50	41.00 ± 1.00	18.46 ± 0.72	0.365 ± 0.0055	-24.5 ± 0.81	99.27 ± 0.64	84.1 ± 1.00
F3	98.3 ± 0.30	55.66 ± 1.15	31.5 ± 1.13	0.334 ± 0.0035	-26.7 ± 0.94	98.79 ± 0.85	69.9 ± 1.40
F4	99.24 ± 0.21	35.00 ± 1.00	17.86 ± 0.55	0.310 ± 0.0020	-62.83 ± 0.75	99.40 ± 0.16	87.00 ± 0.50
F5	98.20± 0.15	59.33 ± 1.52	49.23 ± 0.98	0.401 ± 0.0026	-32.9 ± 0.55	98.38 ± 0.25	69.3 ± 0.50
F6	96.51± 1.30	66.33 ± 1.50	199.3 ± 1.83	0.421 ± 0.0040	-38.96 ± 0.30	97.15 ± 0.37	63.8 ± 0.60
F7	**99.62 ± 0.18**	**20.33 ± 0.57**	**14.73 ± 0.11**	**0.117 ± 0.0011**	**-44.43 ± 0.23**	**99.64 ± 0.12**	**87.7 + 0.60**
F8	94.86 ⊥ 1.12	80.66 ± 0.57	212.8 ± 0.36	0.533 ± 0.0073	-22.13 ± 0.49	95.05 ± 0.63	63.4 ± 1.00

Data expressed as mean ± SD (n = 3)

Table 38. ANOVA for the Model

Response Variables	F-Value	P-Value	R^2	Adjusted R^2	S.D
% Transmittance	17.21	<0.05	0.8959	0.8438	0.6820
Globule size	203.87	<0.05	0.9439	0.9883	8.57
Self emulsification time	33.62	<0.05	0.9916	0.9158	5.90
% Drug release	235.18	<0.05	0.9932	0.9874	0.7392

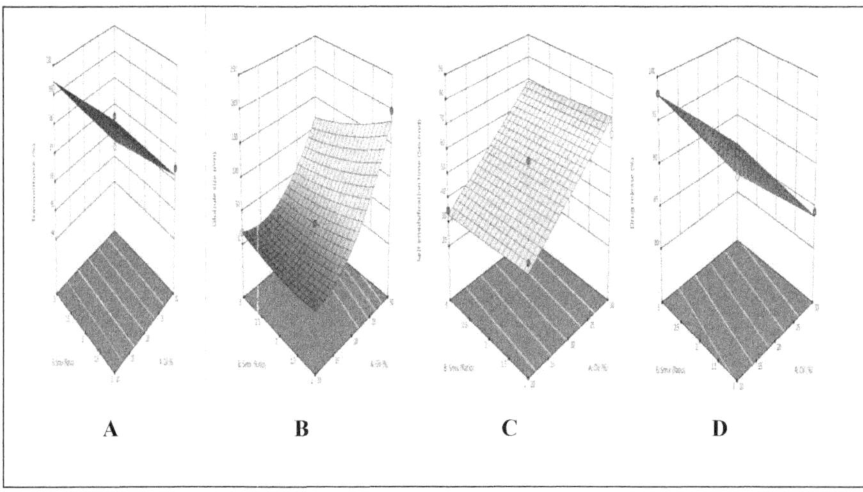

Figure 5. 3D response surface plots for the effect on variables on A) % Transmittance B) Globule size C) Self emulsification time D) % Drug release

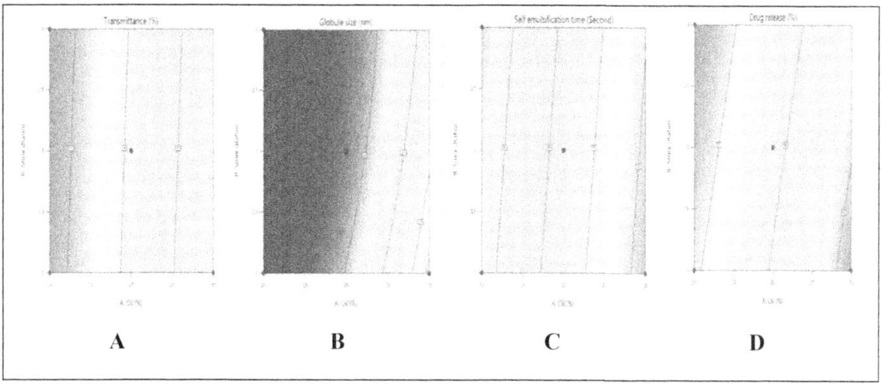

Figure 6. Counter plot for the effect of variables on A) % Transmittance B) globule size C) Self emulsification time D) % Drug release

The CCD model was designed to fit the 2nd order polynomial model using multiple regression analysis equation is as follows,

$Y= b_0 + b_1 X_1+b_2X_2+ b_3X^2_1+ b_4X^2_2+ b_5 X_1X_2$ ... (9)

Where,

Y is the dependent variable (factor),

b_0 is the intercept,

X1and X2 correspond to the studied factors,

b_1-b_5 are the regression coefficients.

Using this polynomial equation and statistical analysis via Design Expert software, the independent and dependent variables were linked. The linear model was used to approximate the responses values of Y1, Y3, and Y4, whereas the quadratic model was used for Y2. The impact of these factors on the responses is linked to the values of the coefficients X1 and X2.

% Transmittance $(Y_1) = + 97.87 - 1.53 X_1 - 0.0741 X_2$ ----------- (10)

Globule size $(Y_2) = + 31.50 + 69.49 X_1 - 13.44 X_2 - 19.11X_1X_2 + 43.19 X^2_1 + 7.31X^2_2$ ---- (11)

Self emulsification time $(Y_3) = + 53.17 + 18.20 X_1 - 1.83 X_2$ -------- (12)

% Drug release $(Y_4) = + 90.95 - 5.81 X_1 + 1.27 X_2$ ----------- (13)

An antagonistic effect was a negative term, whereas a positive sign indicated synergistic reaction. The higher the coefficient, the greater the impact on independent variable has on its response. Table 37 shows that the % transmittance varied from 94.86±1.12% to 99.62±0.18%. According to equation no. 10, the negative coefficient of X_1 indicated that the % transmittance decreased by concentration of oil is increased.

The globule size of the prepared system ranged from 14.73±0.11 nm to 212.8±0.36 nm, as shown in table 37. The emulsion average globule size is important because it impact on drug release and absorption. As per equation 11, positive X_1 coefficient indicated that the globule size increased with the increasing oil concentration.

The self emulsification time for the experimental runs varied from 20.33±0.57 seconds to 80.66±0.57 seconds according to the table 37. As per equation 12 showed that the concentration of oil has a positive effect on self-emulsifying ability.

In the table 37 shows that % drug release of P-L-SEDDS range in between 81.58 ±0.21% and 98.65±0.06%. A reduction of % drug release with an increase in oil concentration was shown by the negative coefficient of X_1 factor as per equation 13. Figure 5 shows 3D response surface plots and figure 6 shows counter plots that support these results.

In this study, desirable responses of optimized formulation were transmittance 99.62%, 14.73 nm globule size, self-emulsification time 20.33 seconds and % drug release 98.65%. Actual photograph of optimized formulation as shown in figure 7.

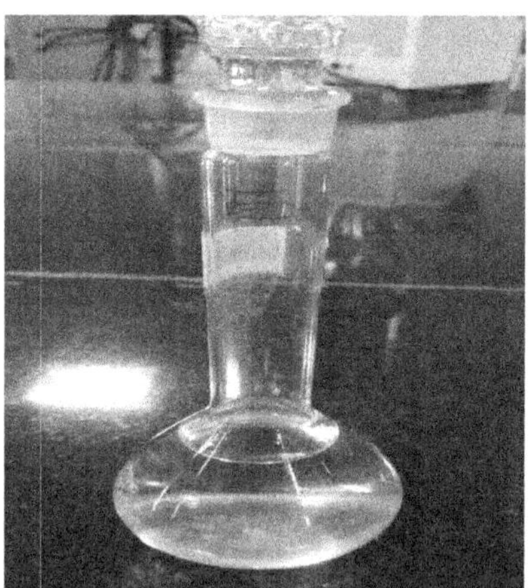

Figure 7. Photograph of optimized liquid SEDDS (F7)

9.8.1. Transmission electron microscopy analysis

The TEM image of optimized liquid formulation (F7) was shown in figure 8. The TEM revealed that particles were almost spherical in shape.

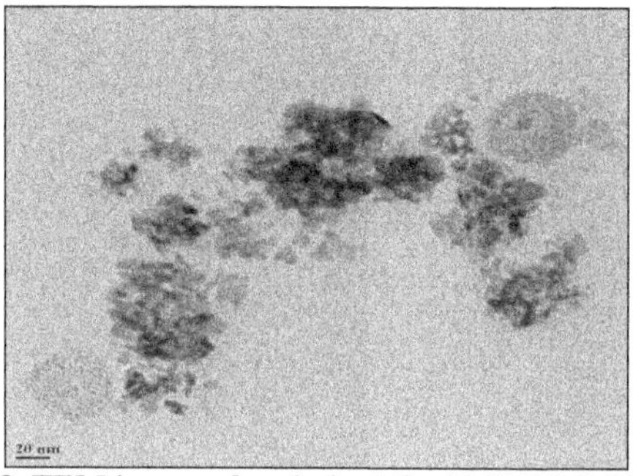

Figure 8. TEM image of optimized liquid SEDDS (F7)

9.8.2. % Transmittance

All experimental runs had transmittance values ranging from 94.86±1.12% to 99.62 ± 0.18% and the % transmittance of the optimized batch was found to be 99.62±0.18%, validating L-SEDDS self-emulsification efficiency.

9.8.3. Globule size determination and polydispersity index

The average globule size of all formulations ranged from 14.73±0.11 nm to 212.8±0.36 nm, which indicated that the nanometric range is for emulsion globules. As shown in figure 9, 14.73± 0.11 nm was the globule size of optimized F7 formulation which was found to be smallest of all other formulations. The polydispersity index optimized F7 formulation was recorded at 0.117±0.0011.

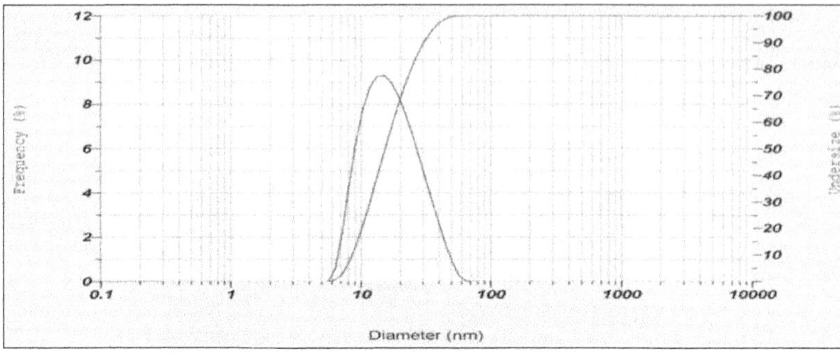

Figure 9. Globule size of optimized F7 formulation

9.8.4. Zeta potential determination

The zeta potential of all SEDDS formulations were negatively charged with values ranging from -22.13 ± 0.49 mV to -44.43 ± 0.23 mV as shown in table 37 and -44.43 mV suggesting a stable system and well separated emulsion globules for an optimized F7 formulation as shown in figure 10.

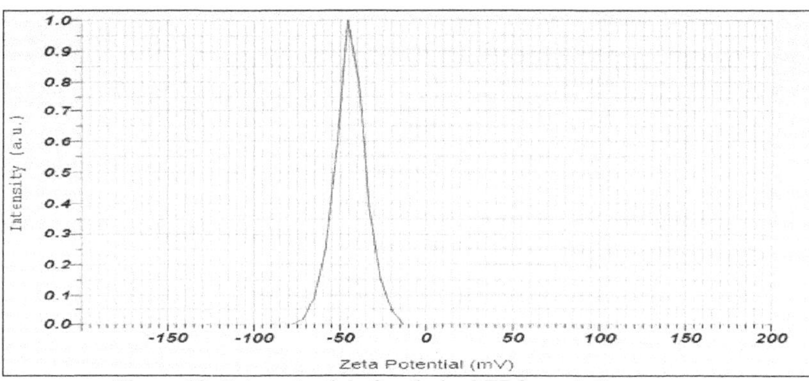

Figure 10. Zeta potential of optimized F7 formulation

9.8.5. Determination of self-emulsification time

The emulsification time findings were obtained in the range of 20.33 ± 0.57 sec. to 80.66 ± 0.57 sec. for all formulations as indicated at table no. 37. For optimized formulation F7 the lowest self-emulsification time was recorded at 20.33 ± 0.57 sec.

9.8.6. Cloud point measurement

The cloud point of optimized P-L-SEDDS F7 formulation was 87.7±0.60°C as shown in table no. 37 indicating that a stable and transparent system will be formed.

9.8.7. Drug content

The drug content of optimized F7 formulation was reported 99.64±0.12%.

9.8.9. *In-vitro* dissolution studies

All SEDDS formulations were subjected to dissolution study and their profiles are presented in figure no. 11 (a) and 11 (b). A maximum drug release of 98.65±0.06% after 30 minutes was shown in the optimized formulation F7. This enhances the solubility and release rate of PZQ with the P-L-SEDDS formulation.

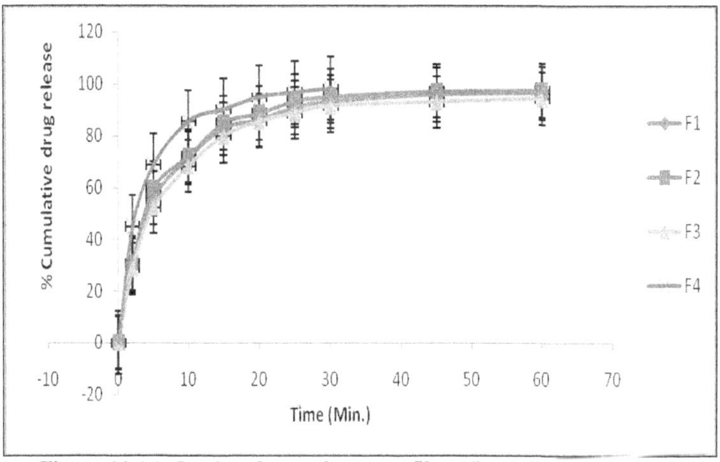

Figure 11 (a). *In-vitro* drug release profile of formulations F1 to F4

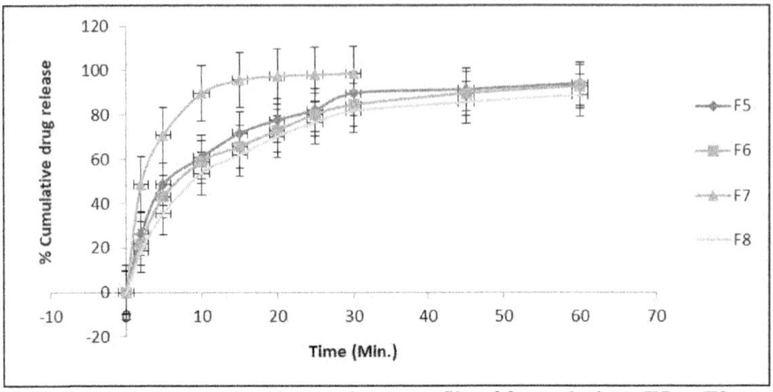

Figure 11 (b). ***In-vitro*** **drug release profile of formulations F5 to F8**

9.8.10. Stability study of F7 liquid SEDDS formulation

The impact of stability condition on the optimized F7 formulation storage for six months was investigated. No significant decrease was seen in % drug content, % transmittance and % drug release as shown in table 39. The results of a stability survey revealed that the optimized F7 formulation retained its stability and remained stable during six months.

Table 39. Stability study data of F7 formulation of liquid SEDDS (at 40°C±2°C/ 75%RH ±5%RH)

Test	After 1 month	After 2 month	After 3 month	After 6 month
Drug content (%)	99.40 ± 0.18	99.16 ± 0.26	98.99± 0.22	97.76 ± 0.14
Transmittance (%)	99.50 ± 0.39	99.42 ± 0.20	98.60 ± 0.15	98.14 ± 0.12
Drug release (%)	98.34 ± 0.22	98.11 ± 0.30	98 ± 0.13	97.46 ± 0.45

Data expressed as mean ± SD (n = 3)

9.9. Anthelmintic activity of earthworms

Six earthworms were collected and transferred immediately to an optimized liquid SEDDS containing petri plate as illustrated in figure 12. The average time taken for paralysis was 1.12±6 minutes and the earthworm died in 1.57±6 minutes. The result showed that anthelmintic activity for earthworms that paralysis and death needed less time when these placed an optimized liquid SEDDS.

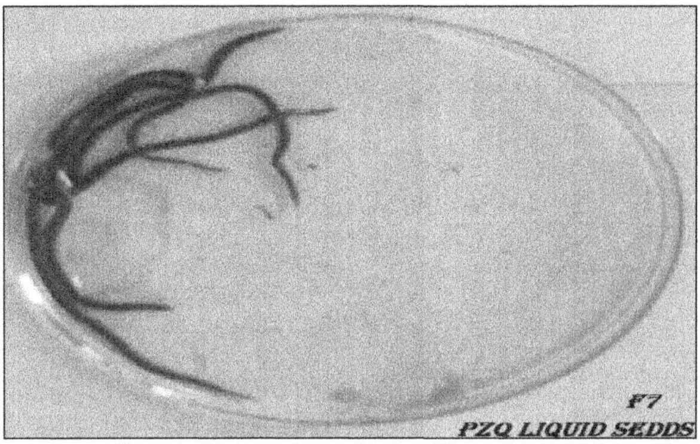

Figure 12. Earthworm in optimized liquid SEDDS (n=6)

9.10. Selection of adsorbent for preparation of S-SEDDS

In order to convert liquid SEDDS into a free-flow powder, two different adsorbents (Aerosil 200 and Neusilin US2) were employed. Neusilin US2 adsorbent needs 100 mg to be turned into free flow powder for optimized liquid SEDDS, while Aerosil 200 needs 120 mg as shown in table 40. Powder characteristics findings were shown in Table 41. From these results, it was found that powder of Neusilin US2 adsorbent has better adsorption capacity and excellent flow properties. A free flow powder from two different adsorbents in a capsule and an *in-vitro* dissolution test was performed. Neusilin US2, a free flow powder based on free-flow granulates with optimum liquid, provides 62.80 % drug release in 5 minutes and 90.83% drug release in 15 minutes as shown in figure 13. As a consequence of the improved adsorption of Neusilin US2 over other research adsorbents. The FTIR, DSC, PXRD and SEM for free flow powder based on Neusilin US2 has been characterized.

Table 40. Adsorbent selection

Formulation	Adsorbent	Amount of Liquid SEDDS (ml)	Amount of adsorbent required to get free flow powder (mg)
A1	Aerosil 200	0.2	120
A2	Neusilin US2	0.2	100

Table 41. Powder characteristics of adsorbents after adsorption of liquid SEDDS

Adsorbents	Parameters					Inference
	Bulk density (gm/ml)	Tapped density (gm/ml)	Carr's index %	Hausner's ratio	Angle of repose(°)	
A1	0.57± 0.025	0.69 ± 0.001	16.44 ± 2.454	1.200 ± 0.034	39.15 ± 0.871	Fair
A2	**0.64 ± 0.015**	**0.71 ± 0.015**	**10.23 ± 0.790**	**1.114 ± 0.009**	**28.53 ± 0.911**	**Excellent**

Data expressed as mean ± SD (n = 3)

The graphical representation of *in-vitro* drug release of Praziquantel from free flow powder of 2 different adsorbents with standard errors is as shown below in figure 13.

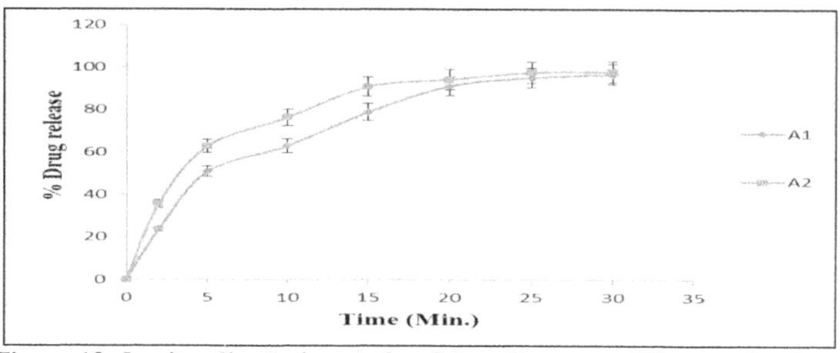

Figure 13. *In-vitro* dissolution study of drug from two different adsorbent

9.10.1. SEM analysis

Scanning electron microscopy reveals the morphology of solid SEDDS. Micrographs of Solid SEDDS shows liquid SEDDS adsorbed onto the surface of Neusilin US2 particles which shown in fig. 14. Since the formulation process involved facilitating adsorption through physical mixing, partially covered Neusilin US2 is also visible in the field of vision.

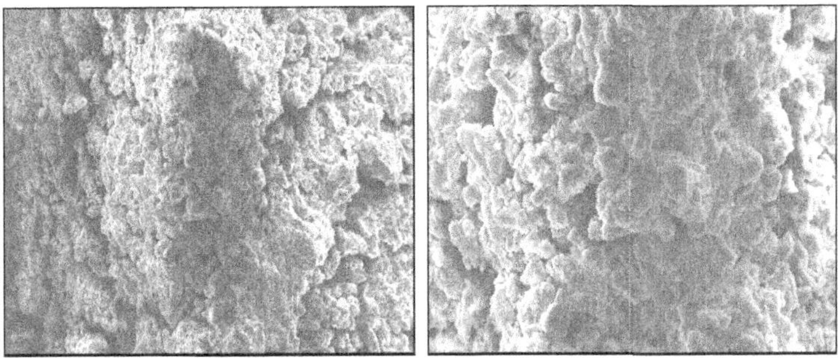

Figure 14. SEM images of solid SEDDS

9.10.2. DSC studies

DSC is a useful technique that gives an insight into the melting and crystallization behavior of crystalline materials like S-SEDDS. The DSC thermogram of pure drug PZQ and Solid SEDDS are as shown in Figure 15 (A) & (B). Pure drug substance shows a sharp endothermic peak at 141^{0}C which shows the highly crystalline behavior of drug. Whereas, no peak was observed in S-SEDDS formulation which shows the change in melting behavior of drug and inhibition of crystallization following granulation using lipid surfactants.

.

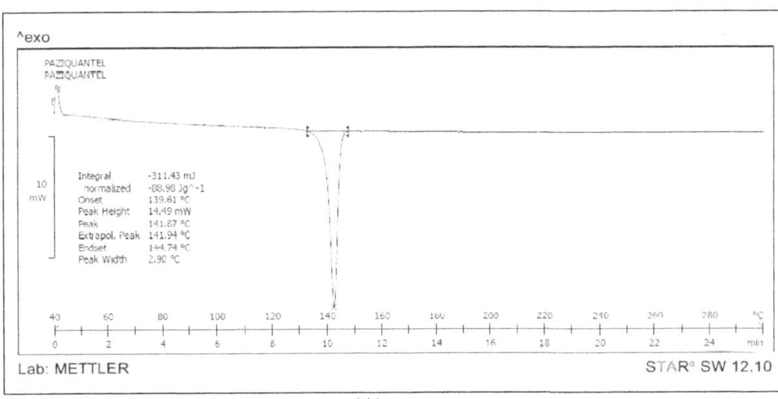

(A)

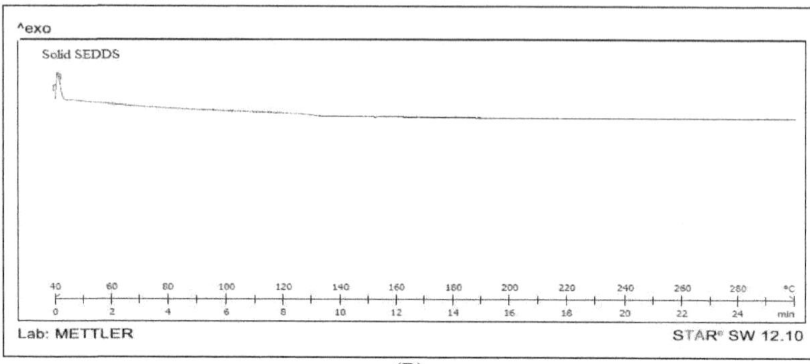

(B)

Figure 15. DSC thermogram of (A) Praziquantel (B) Solid SEDDS Powder

9.10.3. FT-IR Spectroscopy

To check computability of the PZQ with selected excipient, FT-IR was carried out. There was no significant difference between the drug wave number (cm-1) and the optimized solid SEDDS powder. The FTIR analysis as shown in figure 16 (A) & (B) show similar spectra of PZQ drug and the corresponding physical mixtures indicating the formation of hydrogen bonding between the components of the formulation, as previously observed for PZQ. These results show the absence of strong interactions between PZQ and S-SEDDS.

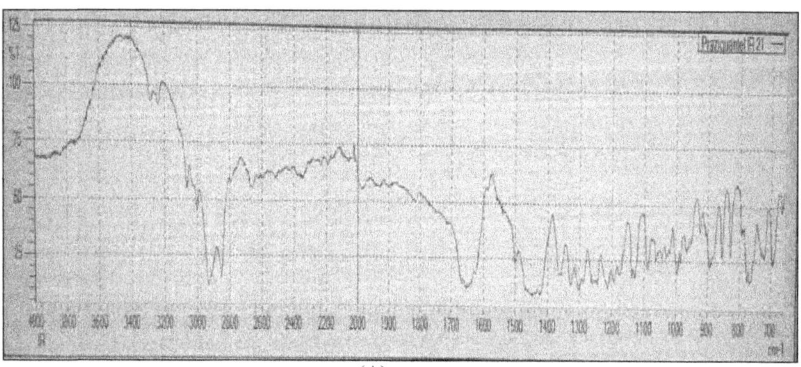

(A)

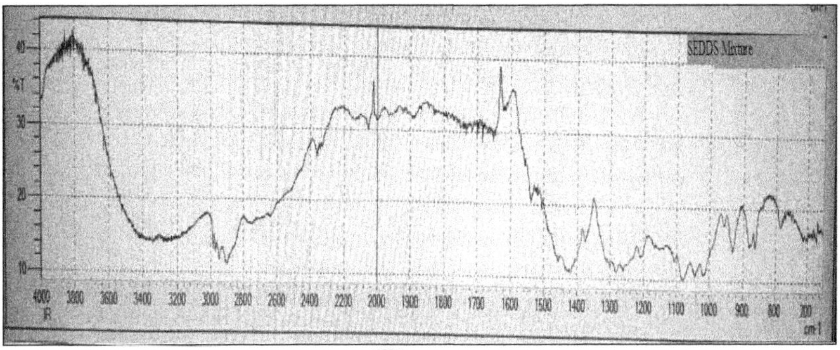

(B)

Figure 16. Infrared spectra of (A) Praziquantel (B) S-SEDDS mixture

9.10.4. X-ray diffraction (XRD) analysis

The XRD pattern as shown in figure no. 17 (A) and (B). XRD studies of Praziquantel pure drug showed several sharp peak at 5-25$^0\theta$ indicating crystalline nature as shown in figure 17 (A). Crystalline substances create sharp XRD diffraction patterns, whereas non crystalline or amorphous substances create hard distinguished and broad patterns. The PZQ in the S-SEDDS showed no sharp peaks which proved that the drug was molecularly dispersed in the oil-Smix which retained its integrity even after adsorption as shown in figure 17 (B).

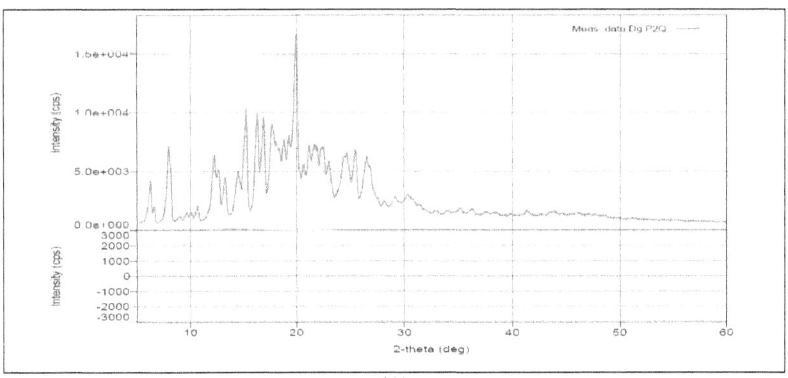

(A)

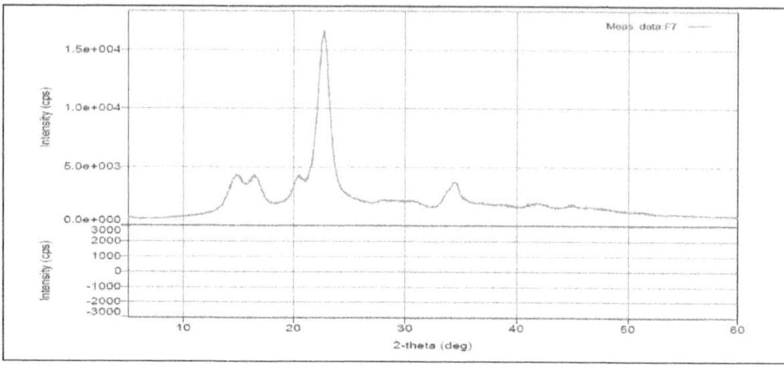

(B)

Figure 17. XRD spectra of (A) Praziquantel (B) Optimized S-SEDDS

9.10.5. Evaluation of S-SEDDS tablets

Table 42 shows the assessment criteria for T1 to T9 batches. The hardness of tablets was ranged from 3.53±0.57 kg/cm^2 to 3.83±152 kg/cm^2. These are all tablets have very good mechanical strength. These tablets have a thickness of 2.60±0.152 mm to 3.13±0.208 mm. The friability of all formulations was found to be less than 1.0 % and was in the range of 0.13 ±0.026% to 0.67± 0.225 % indicating a good mechanical resistance of tablets. The uniformity of weight was found to be in the range of 249.00±1.000 mg to 251.33±1.527 mg. The % drug content of tablets was found to be between 95.53±0.894% to 99.71±0.098%. All these characteristics were verified acceptable and compliance with the Praziquantel tablet criteria. The disintegration time for batch T3 was found to be 10 sec. Compared to previous batches; this tablet has the quickest disintegration time. *In vitro* drug release results for T1 to T9 batches are shown in figures 18 (a) and 18 (b). While all batches to produce 56.79% to 73.78% of drug release after 5 minutes and 73.78% drug release of T3 batch in 5 minutes at a higher rate than the other batches. Therefore, the batch T3 was regarded as the optimized batch and used for further research.

Table 42. Evaluation parameters for Praziquantel S-SEDDS tablets

Formulation code	Hardness (kg/cm2)	Thickness (mm)	Uniformity of Weight (mg)	Friability (%)	Disintegration time (sec.)	Drug Content (%)*
T1	3.56±0.057	2.83±0.057	251.00±1.000	0.33±0.040	15.66±1.527	98.89±0.375
T2	3.66±0.115	3.13±0.208	249.33±0.577	0.20±0.035	12.33±0.577	99.34±0.110
T3	**3.53±0.057**	**2.90±0.100**	**250.00±1.000**	**0.13±0.026**	**10.00±1.000**	**99.71±0.098**
T4	3.80±0.100	2.60±0.152	251.33±1.527	0.39±0.057	38.33±1.527	97.48±0.490
T5	3.60±0.100	2.93±0.152	249.00±1.000	0.36±0.124	29.33±0.152	97.84±0.444
T6	3.76±0.152	2.86±0.115	250.00.±1.732	0.28±0.020	25.00±1.000	98.65±0.502
T7	3.73±0.152	2.76±0.057	250.66±1.527	0.67±0.225	42.00±1.00	95.53±0.894
T8	3.70±0.173	2.73±0.057	250.33±1.527	0.49±0.155	31.66±1.154	97.06±0.456
T9	3.83±0.152	2.66±0.115	249.66±1.732	0.42±0.217	26.33±1.527	97.33±1.176

Data expressed as mean ± SD (n = 3)

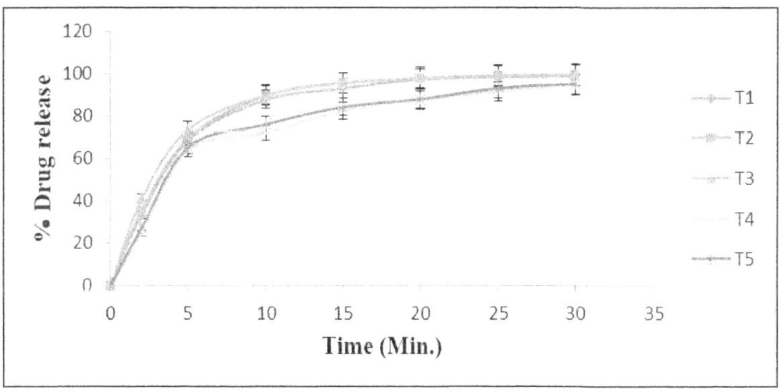

Figure 18 (a). *In-vitro* drug release profile of formulations T1 to T5

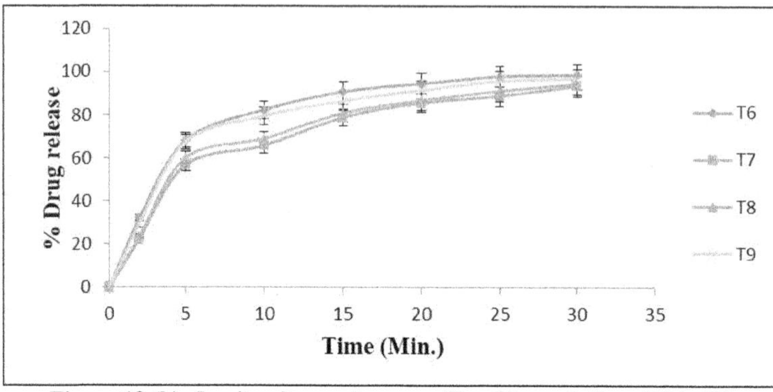

Figure 18 (b). *In-vitro* drug release profile of formulations T6 to T9

9.10.6. Comparison of *In-Vitro* dissolution study of optimized batch T3 with marketed formulation (Distoside Tablet)

In-vitro drug release of optimized T3 batch was compared to the marketed tablet, i.e. (M). In 15 minutes, batch T3 shows 95.54% of drug release in 0.1 N HCl containing 2% SLS, whereas marketed formulation shows 53.86% of drug releases by 15 minutes as shown in figure 19. These results clearly demonstrate the solubility enhances and dissolution was increased of S-SEDDS Praziquantel tablet.

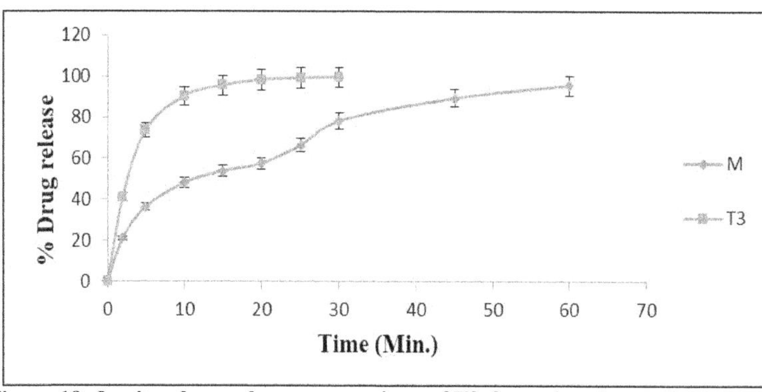

Figure 19. *In-vitro* drug release comparison of T3 & marketed sample (M)

9.10.7. Similarity Factor

Similarity factor was obtained after comparison of dissolution profile of optimized formulation T3 and marketed formulation. Comparison of drug release profile of test (T3 Optimized formulation) and reference (Marketed formulation) as shown in figure 19.

Similarity Factor *f2*:- 54.45.

The value of *f2* value was found to be between 50 to 100. Hence, it indicated similarity between the dissolution profiles of reference and test products.

9.10.8. Accelerated stability studies

An accelerated stability analysis (40°±2°C /75%±5% RH) on the optimized T3 batch has been carried out for duration of six months. These tablets are not significantly modified, as are the disintegration time, globule size, Zeta potential, % drug content and % drug release as shown in table 43.

Table 43. Evaluation parameters of optimized formulation T3 during stability study

Time (In Months)	Parameters				
	Disintegration time (sec.)	Globule size (nm) ± S.D.	Zeta potential (mv) ± S.D.	Drug content (%)	Drug release (%)
0	10.00±1.00	83.3±0.1	-39.56±0.15	99.78±0.085	99.56±0.09
1 M	10.33±1.52	83.5±0.15	-39.23±0.20	98.39±0.82	98.63±0.66
2 M	11.66±1.15	84±0.55	-39.00±0.1	97.80±0.67	98.12±0.59
3 M	12.00±1.00	84.1±0.1	-39.13±0.35	97.42±1.11	97.40±0.48
6 M	12.66±0.57	84.4±0.25	-39.16±0.30	96.83±0.79	96.95±0.14

Mean ± S.D., n=3

9.11. Taste masking evaluation by human panel

The sensory scores reported of a human panel in taste masking study seen in Table 44. Tables reveal that the resin complexes with Praziquantel have been tasted and scored. The Praziquantel resin complex flavour score indicated a lack of bitterness in comparison with Praziquantel (3.00±0.000). The pure material cannot be maintained in the mouth for more than 30 seconds. The flavour of the resin complex is more maskable (1.00±0.000). Sweet taste of T3 optimized batch tablet was due to the existence of Aspartame and Mannitol in formulation.

Table 44. Taste masking evaluation parameters

Sr. No.	Description	Volunteer Score						Mean score ± S.D
		I	II	III	IV	V	VI	
1	Praziquantel	3	3	3	3	3	3	3.00±0.000
2	Praziquantel-Doshion P-544 DS resin Complex	1	1	1	1	1	1	1.00±0.000

Given that the taste evaluation procedure was a "swirl and spit," there was no need for ethical clearance. Until spitting a flavour, volunteers can place it on their tongue and move it about one minute in their mouth to get a flavour. The medicine is not provided or drunk. PZQ is an anthelmintic medicine. PZQ was found to be safe after the "swirl and spit" analysis. As a matter of fact, a taste evaluation of the dosage shape was done on healthy and adult human participants in relation to the efficiency of medicines in children. For the production of the final part, PZQ was inserted into the Doshion Polymer P-544 DS. As PZQ was reduced at salivary pH, the bitter taste of test samples stored in the oral cavity for 1 minute could not be detected by humans. The inclusion of Aspartame and Mannitol, the final result has a sweet flavour. The results show that Doshion P-544 DS is a sophisticated polymer masking that significantly reduces the bitter taste of PZQ.

9.12. BIOANALYTICAL METHOD DEVELOPMENT

9.12.1. Mobile Phase

Acetonitrile-Methanol-Water in ratio of 50:10:40 v/v showed maximum extraction and recovery above 90.00% at a concentration range 100.0–1000.0 ng/mL; thus used as mobile phase.

9.12.2. Selection of Mobile Phase

In order to find the suitable mobile phase for the bioanalytical method moving extraction with different solvents were selected. Extraction was performed with methanol, acetonitrile and acetonitrile with 0.1% o-phthaldialdehyde.

Extraction of Praziquantel with different concentrations as shown in below tables

Table 45. % Recovery with Methanol at 100 ng/mL

Concentration (ng/mL)	AUC	Conc. Found	Recovery %
100	71.45	85.61759777	85.6175978
100	70.65	84.81759777	84.8175978
100	69.12	83.28759777	83.2875978

Table 46. % Recovery with Methanol at 500 ng/mL

Concentration (ng/mL)	AUC	Conc. Found	Recovery %
500	385.67	399.8375978	79.9675196
500	387.6	401.7675978	80.3535196
500	379.03	393.1975978	78.6395196

Table 47. % Recovery with Methanol at 1000 ng/mL

Concentration (ng/mL)	AUC	Conc. Found	Recovery %
1000	846.11	860.2775978	86.0277598
1000	833.26	847.4275978	84.7427598
1000	821.76	835.9275978	83.5927598

Table 48. % Recovery with Acetonitrile:Methanol at 100ng/mL (60:40 v/v)

Concentration (ng/mL)	AUC	Conc. Found	Recovery %
100	73.87	88.03759777	88.0375978
100	72.35	86.51759777	86.5175978
100	71.89	86.05759777	86.0575978

Table 49. % Recovery with Acetonitrile:Methanol at 500ng/mL (60:40 v/v)

Concentration (ng/mL)	AUC	Conc. Found	Recovery %
500	396.23	410.3975978	82.0795196
500	384.11	398.2775978	79.6555196
500	396.46	410.6275978	82.1255196

Table 50. % Recovery with Acetonitrile:Methanol at 1000 ng/mL (60:40 v/v)

Concentration (ng/mL)	AUC	Conc. Found	Recovery %
1000	856.11	870.2775978	87.0277598
1000	864.24	878.4075978	87.8407598
1000	846.32	860.4875978	86.0487598

Table 51. % Recovery with Acetonitrile:Methanol:Water at 100ng/mL (50:10:40 v/v)

Concentration (ng/mL)	AUC	Conc. Found	Recovery %
100	76.56	90.72759777	90.7275978
100	77.11	91.27759777	91.2775978
100	76.89	91.05759777	91.0575978

Table 52. % Recovery with Acetonitrile:Methanol:Water at 500 ng/mL (50:10:40 v/v)

Concentration (ng/mL)	AUC	Conc. Found	Recovery %
500	438.11	452.2775978	90.4555196
500	437.09	451.2575978	90.2515196
500	436.77	450.9375978	90.1875196

Table 53. % Recovery with Acetonitrile:Methanol:Water at 1000 ng/mL (50:10:40 v/v)

Concentration (ng/mL)	AUC	Conc. Found	Recovery %
1000	899.21	913.3775978	91.3377598
1000	897.56	911.7275978	91.1727598
1000	890.17	904.3375978	90.4337598

Using chromatographic analysis by using 0.45 μm membrane filter paper, the mobile phases of Acetonitrile-Methanol-Water (50:10:40 v/v) have been filtered. The flow rates were at 1.0 ml/min for mobile phases and at 217 nm eluent detected. Inject 2 mL volume with a 10 minute running time.

9.12.3. Linearity

To verify the linearity of the method, a standard solution was prepared by using Praziquantel in 100 ng/ml-1500 ng/ml. After injection, peak regions were used to construct the calibration curves against the concentration. The coefficients of correlation of all these seven analytes were 0.999 as shown in graph 8. The findings are shown in Table 54.

Table 54. Linearity concentration Vs Area Under Curve

Concentration (ng/ml)	AUC
10	4.78
50	23.44

100	74.21
500	418.55
1000	892.34
1300	1134.23
1500	1345.67
r2	0.999

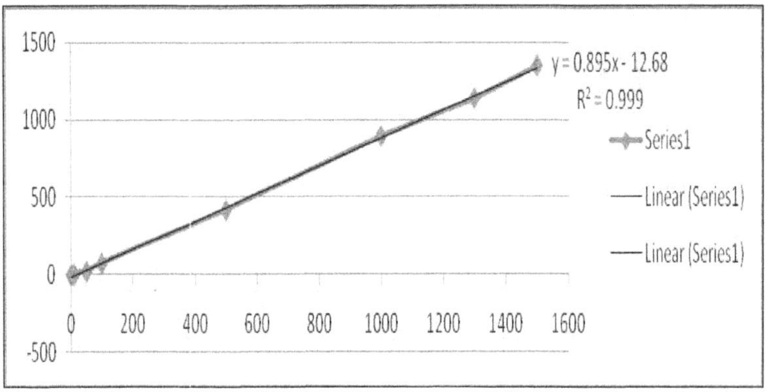

Graph 8. Linearity graph of PZQ

9.12.4. Pharmacokinetic data analysis

Plasma concentration *vs.* time data of Praziquantel was analyzed by Pk solver version 2.0 to derive various pharmacokinetic parameters, *viz.*, $AUC_{0\text{-}t}$, $AUC_{0\text{-}\infty}$, C_{max}, t_{max} and $t\frac{1}{2}$.

Table 55. Summary Table- Input Variable

Time In Hr	Time in Minutes	Plasma Drug Conc. Mcg/ml	Log Plasma Drug Conc. Mcg/ml
0	0	0	0
0.15	15	81.23	1.909716453
0.5	30	156.34	2.194070108
1	60	354.21	2.549260818
2	120	591.24	2.771763808
4	240	432.27	2.635755096

8	480	341.1	2.532881719
12	720	234.98	2.371030899
20	1200	115.23	2.061565562
24	1440	88.14	1.945173046

Table 56. Summary Table- Output

Time	Conc.	ln(C)	AUC	AUMC
0	0	0	0	0
0.15	81.23	4.39728464	6.09225	0.9138375
0.5	156.34	5.05203312	47.667	16.725875
1	354.21	5.86988996	175.3045	124.820875
2	591.24	6.38222203	648.0295	893.165875
4	432.27	6.06905039	1671.5395	3804.72588
8	341.1	5.83217569	3218.2795	12720.4859
12	234.98	5.4595004	4370.4395	23817.6059
20	115.23	4.74693013	5771.2795	44315.0459
24	88.14	4.47892646	6178.0195	53154.9659

Table 57. Pharmacokinetic Calculation Results

Parameter	Marketed Formulation	T3 Formulation
AUC (h ng/ml)	6177.90±1.73	13261.84±1.50
$t^{1/2}$ (h)	1.05 ±0.33	1.30±0.21
Cmax (ng/ml)	147.92±2.08	260.66±1.14
Tmax (h)	2.00±0.50	1.20±0.20
MRT (h)	11.74±1.13	13.47±0.55
Cl (ml h^{-1} g^{-1})	0.028±0.002	0.055±0.001

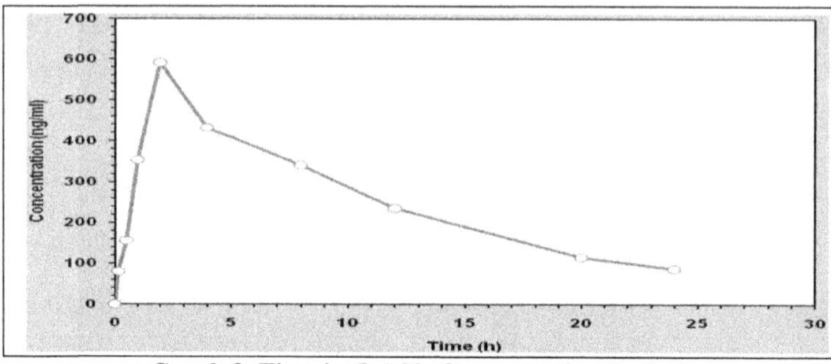

Graph 9. Time in (hr) Vs Concentration (µg/ml)

9.12.5. Validation of method

In accordance with the ICH guidelines for system suitability, specificity, accuracy, linearity, precision and robustness, the proposed bioanalytical method HPLC for Praziquantel was tested.

9.12.5.1. Linearity range

Table 58 shows the ratio of peak areas of Praziquantel with the diazepam (Internal Standard) at varying levels of Praziquantel in plasma. Chromatographic responses were shown to be linear in an analysis range of 100.0-1500.0 ng/ml, with a regression coefficient (r^2) of 0.999, indicating that the technique was reproducible. For the linear regression equation $Y=0.895x - 12.68$ was calculated.

Table 58. The ratio of peak areas of Praziquantel to Praziquantel IS at various concentrations

Concentration of Praziquantel (ng/mL)	peak area		Peak area of the chromatogram Ratio
	Praziquantel	Diazepam IS	
10	4.78	4.33	1.103926097
50	23.44	22.98	1.020017406
100	74.21	74.53	0.995706427
500	418.55	416.22	2.725073279
1000	892.34	895.09	1.50339072

1300	1134.23	1124.67	1.008500271
1500	1345.67	1347.81	0.998412239

9.12.5.2. System Suitability

The HPLC system was injected in six replicates with standard Praziquantel solutions of 100 ng/mL. The standard solutions have been identified by using chromatographic functions such as Rt values and peak areas and the results showed that the system is appropriate for analysis as shown in table 59.

Table 59. System suitability Parameters

Drug	Retention Time (Rt)	Peak Area
Praziquantel	6.41	2245311

9.12.5.3. Precision and accuracy

Precision and accuracy of the method for the estimation of Praziquantel in rat plasma. $y = 0.895x - 12.68$.

Table 60. Intra-day precision (Day 1)

Concentration (ng/mL)	Intra-day precision			RSD %	Accuracy %
100	79.24	91.92	102.7039	2.13	102.7039106
500	448.91	461.59	515.743	1.0916	103.1486034
1000	891.56	904.24	1010.324	1.1166	101.0324022

Table 61. Intra-day precision (Day 2)

Concentration (ng/mL)	Intra-day precision			RSD %	Accuracy %
100	81.39	94.07	105.1061	2.13	105.1061453
500	449.04	461.72	515.8883	1.0916	103.1776536
1000	892.33	905.01	1011.184	1.1166	101.1184358

Table 62. Intra-day precision (Day 3)

Concentration (ng/mL)	Intra-day precision			RSD %	Accuracy %
100	78.99	91.67	102.4246	2.13	102.424581
500	447.21	459.89	513.8436	1.0916	102.7687151
1000	891.11	903.79	1009.821	1.1166	100.9821229

Table 63. Inter-day precision

Concentration (ng/mL)	Inter-day precision			RSD %	Accuracy %
100	78.68	91.36	102.0782	2.705	102.0782123
500	449.91	462.59	516.8603	1.1748	103.372067
1000	891.44	904.12	1010.19	1.212	101.0189944

Table 64. Intra-day Accuracy

Concentration (ng/mL)	Concentration (ng/mL)	Concentration (ng/mL)	Average	Standard Deviation	Relative standard Deviation
100.56	100.11	100.24	112	0.2315887	0.206775639
500.87	500.31	500.9	559.6648	0.3323151	0.059377525
1000.81	1000.78	1000.25	1117.598	0.3150132	0.028186637

Table 65. Inter-day Accuracy

Concentration (ng/mL)	Concentration (ng/mL)	Concentration (ng/mL)	Average	Standard Deviation	Relative standard Deviation
100.39	100.22	100.11	111.8547	0.1410674	0.126116559
500.91	500.8	500.17	558.8492	0.399291	0.071448803
1000.51	1000.09	1000.23	1117.575	0.2138535	0.01913549

9.12.5.4. Specificity

Blank, standard and samples of Praziquantel solutions were injected into duplicates at 100 ng/mL concentration. For all solutions, the chromatograms obtained were compared for the specificity of the technique. Standard and sample solutions were generated after comparison of the chromatograms of blank solutions. The obtained chromatograms show that there are no co-eluting peaks throughout the corresponding retention period (Rt- 6.41). Therefore, the method was found to be specific.

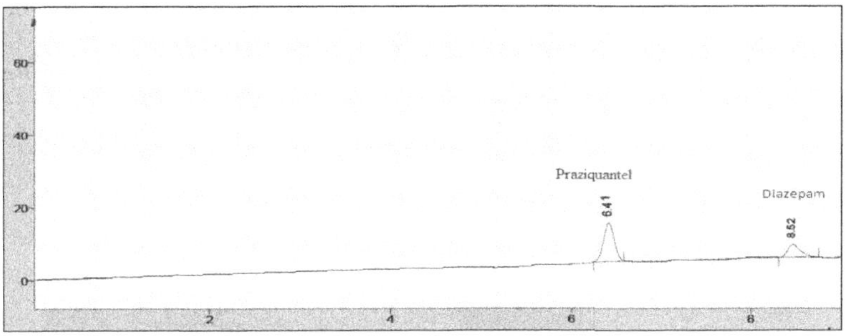

Figure 20. Chromatogram of STD Praziquantel and Diazepam IS solution

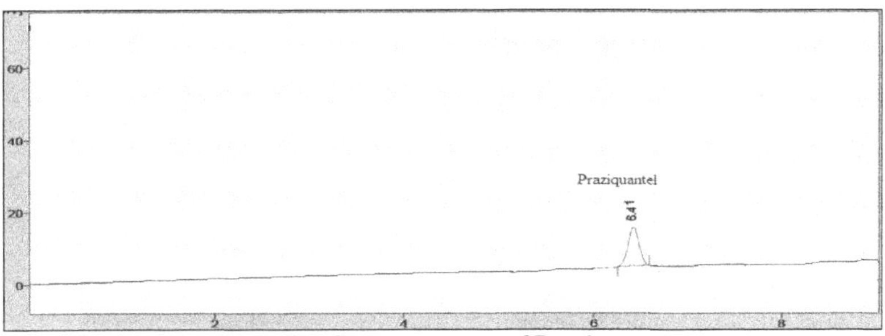

Figure 21. Chromatogram of Praziquantel

9.12.5.5. Method precision

The samples solutions of Praziquantel having concentrations 100 µg/ml were injected in 6 replicates and analyzed for drug content. The % assay for both the analytes were calculated and results were expressed in terms of % Relative Standard Deviation as shown in table 66.

Table 66. Method Precision

Sampling Sr. Number	Praziquantel % Assay
1	91.23
2	92.01
3	91.11
4	91.06
5	92.44
6	91.05
Mean % Assay	91.48
Standard Deviation	0.78
% Relative Standard Deviation	0.65

The average % assay for Praziquantel was determined and the % RSD values were found to be within the acceptable criteria <2.0%.

9.12.5.6. Robustness

The effects of changes in chromatographic conditions were determined conferring to ICH guidelines to establish robustness of the bioanalytical method. The change in the flow rate, mobile phase composition of Praziquantel was considered. The retention time of Praziquantel was determined and % RSD for each changing chromatographic condition was calculated.

Table 67. Robustness parameters

Sr. No	Parameters	Established Parameters	Changes in the parameters
1	Flow	1.0 ml/min	1.1 ml/min
2	**Mobile phase composition (Acetonitrile:Methanol:Water)**	50:10:40%	60:10:30%

The chromatographic analysis of Praziquantel was not influenced by changes in flow rate and mobile phase composition as shown in Table 68. For Praziquantel standard solutions, the % RSD of peak-area responses was found to be less than 2.0%. Therefore, the method was found to be robust.

Table 68. Robustness for Praziquantel

Robustness parameter		**% RSD for Praziquantel**
Flow (mL/min.)	1.0	0.27
	1.1	0.28
Mobile phase composition (Acetonitrile:Methanol:Water)	50:10:40%	0.22
	60:10:30%	0.39

10. SUMMARY

- The drug was characterized by determination of melting point, FT-IR, DSC and PXRD. It was confirmed that the received sample was PZQ.
- Based on solubility study and emulsification ability study following components were screened for the formulation of P-L-SEDDS.
    - ✓ Oil – Capmul MCM
    - ✓ Surfactant – Cremophore RH40
    - ✓ Co-surfactant – PEG400
- From the above components, further selection of the surfactant and co-surfactant and working concentration ranges of these components of L-SEDDS was done by using pseudo ternary phase diagrams. The SEDDS developed here in were evaluated for thermodynamic stability study, dispersibility study, robustness to dilution, % transmittance, globule size and self emulsification time. The pseudo ternary phase diagrams suggested the following for effective formulation of L-SEDDS.
    - Oil concentration (Capmul MCM): 10% - 30%
    - Smix ratio (Cremophore RH40:PEG400): 1:1 to 3:1
- The optimization of the P-L-SEDDS formulation was done by CCD incorporating 2 independent variables viz. oil concentration and Smix ratio; 4 dependent variables viz. % transmittance, globule size, self emulsification time and % drug release.
- It was observed that,
    - As oil amount increased then % transmittance is decrease.
    - An increase in oil concentration then increased globule size
    - As indicated positive influence of oil concentration on the self emulsification ability.
    - An increase in oil concentration then decreased % drug release.
- Eight experimental runs were suggested by the CCD design to fit the second order polynomial model using multiple regression analysis.
- The optimized batch had % transmittance, globule size, self-emulsification time and % drug release of 99.62% ±0.18, 14.73±0.11 nm, 20.33±0.57 sec. and 98.65% ±0.06. Its zeta potential, polydispersity index and % drug content were 44.43±0.23 mv, 0.117±0.0011 and 99.64 % ±0.12. The cloud point of optimized P-L-SEDDS

formulation was much higher than 87°C indicating that a stable and transparent system will be formed.

- Anthelmintic activity for earthworms showed that paralysis and death needed less time for these earthworms when placed in an optimized liquid SEDDS.
- The optimized P-L-SEDDS was converted into P-S-SEDDS by adsorption on the Neusilin US2.
- The optimized P-S-SEDDS was characterized for flow properties by measuring the Bulk density, Tap density, Carr's index, Hausner's ratio and Angle of repose; values for these tests were 0.64 ± 0.015, 0.71 ± 0.015 , 10.23% ± 0.790, 1.114 ± 0.009 and 28.53° ± 0.911 respectively. Neusilin US2, a free flow powder based on free-flow granulates with optimum liquid, provides 62.80 % drug release in 5 minutes and 90.83% drug release in 15 minutes. The FT-IR study showed the characteristic absorption peaks of PZQ were retained in P-S-SEDDS formulation without any additional peaks. DSC thermogram of pure PZQ showed a sharp endothermic peak at 140^0C which was absent in blank S-SEDDS. The PXRD diffractogram of the PZQ showed characteristic high intensity diffraction peaks at 2θ values of $5\text{-}25^0$ θ indicating crystalline nature. PZQ loaded solid SEDDS revealed that peak of mixture was observed at $15\text{-}25^0\theta$.
- HPLC method for determination of PZQ in plasma was validated and used for further *in vivo* study.
- The pharmacokinetic profile of the optimized P-S-SEDDS tablet was studied in comparison with marketed tablet. The AUC was found to be 13261.84±1.50 ng.h/ml and 6177.90±1.73 ng.h/ml for optimized S-SEDDS tablet T3 batch and marketed tablet respectively. The peak drug concentration (Cmax) of optimized S-SEDDS tablet T3 batch was approximately 1.76 fold higher than marketed tablet.
- The optimized S-SEDDS tablets (T3) were found to be chemically and physically stable for 6 months.
- The optimized S-SEDDS tablet batch enhanced the solubility and oral bioavailability of PZQ.

11. CONCLUSION

In this present study, P-L-SEDDS and P-S-SEDDS were developed to improve the bioavailability of PZQ. The stable and uniform nano-sized P-L-SEDDS and P-S-SEDDS were formed. P-L-SEDDS and P-S-SEDDS were characterized by various *in vitro* and *in vivo* studies. The results of the *in vitro* studies pointed out that the incorporation of Praziquantel in a liquid SEDDS and S-SEDDS tablets enhanced its solubility and release rate. Anthelmintic action on earthworms was significant in the optimized P-L-SEDDS (F7). This may lead to the development of P-L-SEDDS as a effective for worm infection treatment.

The optimized S-SEDDS formulation T3 showed minimum disintegration time and maximum drug release. *In-vitro* drug release of the optimized batch T3 was higher than as compared to a marketed conventional tablet (M). *In vivo* pharmacokinetic investigation in rats, demonstrated significantly higher AUC by the developed optimized S-SEDDS tablet. The optimized S-SEDDS tablets (T3) were found to be chemically and physically stable for 6 months. All these findings concluded that the developed P-L-SEDDS and P-S-SEDDS improved solubility, oral bioavailability, and therapeutic applicability anthelmintic agent of PZQ. Today, PZQ remains the drug of choice for all forms of schistosomiasis occurring in humans, because of its high efficacy, low toxicity and ease of single, oral administration compared to the other medicines. Thus it can be concluded that S-SEDDS would be a promising dosage form in the prevention of worm infections for pediatric patients.

12. FUTURE SCOPE

- The developed S-SEDDS is a useful solid platform technology for improving solubility and oral bioavailability of PZQ.

9 781805 252009

Printed by BoD™in Norderstedt, Germany